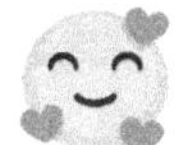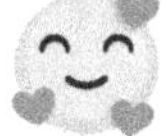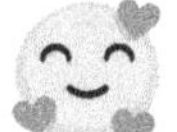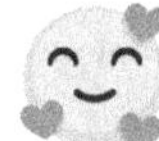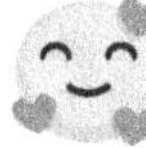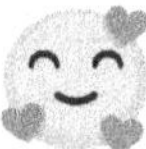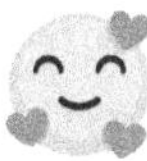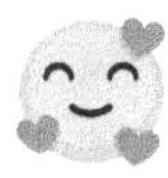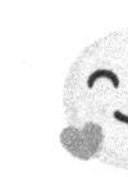

2. Pizza (various toppings)

 Prep Time :   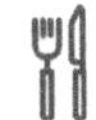 Cook Time :   Servings :

Let's do that and fill in the time here

Write 5 friends with whom you want to share this dish

....
....
....
....
....

Is this dish easy or difficult for you to make?

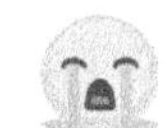 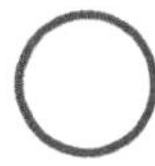 ◯   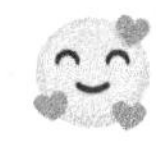 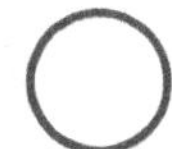 ◯

INGREDIENTS

- 1 pre-made pizza crust or flatbread
- 1 cup marinara or pizza sauce
- 2 cups shredded mozzarella cheese
- Assorted toppings (choose 2-3):
  - Pepperoni
  - Cooked Italian sausage
  - Diced bell peppers
  - Sliced mushrooms
  - Diced onions
  - Black olives
  - Pineapple chunks

1. Preheat the oven to 400°F.

2. Spread the pizza sauce evenly over the crust or flatbread, leaving a small border around the edges.

3. Sprinkle the shredded mozzarella cheese over the sauce.

4. Add your desired toppings, distributing them evenly over the cheese.

5. Bake the pizza for 12-15 minutes, until the cheese is melted and bubbly and the crust is lightly golden.

6. Let the pizza cool for 5 minutes, then slice and serve.

Tips:
- Use pre-shredded cheese to make it even easier.
- Encourage teens to get creative with their topping choices.
- Serve with a side salad or veggie sticks for a more balanced meal.
- For a personal-sized pizza, use an individual-sized flatbread or English muffin.

This recipe is simple, customizable, and perfect for young teens to make themselves or with a little adult supervision. Enjoy!

Did you have fun cooking this dish?

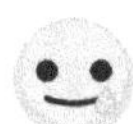  ◯    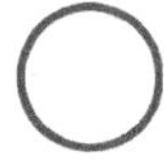 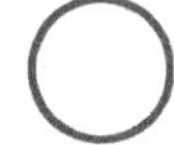 ◯

How would you rate this dish?

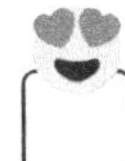 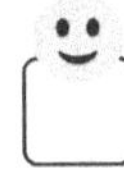 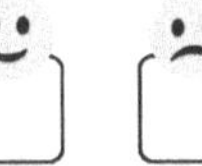  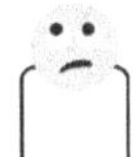 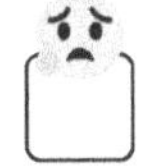

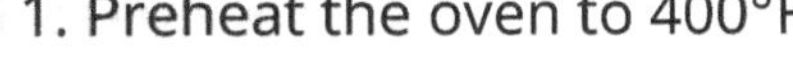

3. Chicken nuggets

Let's do that and fill in the time here  Prep Time :   Cook Time :   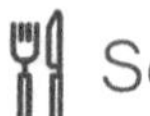 Servings :

Write 5 friends with whom you want to share this dish
....
....
....
....
....

INGREDIENTS

- 1 lb boneless, skinless chicken breasts, cut into 1-inch pieces
- 1 cup panko breadcrumbs
- 1/2 cup all-purpose flour
- 2 eggs, beaten
- 1/2 tsp salt
- 1/4 tsp black pepper
- 1/4 tsp garlic powder
- Cooking spray

Is this dish easy or difficult for you to make?

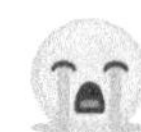 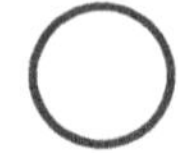 ◯   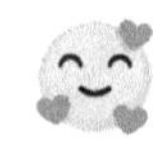 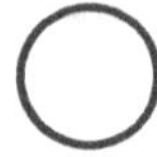 ◯

1. Preheat the oven to 400°F. Line a baking sheet with parchment paper or a silicone baking mat.

2. Set up a breading station with three shallow dishes:
   - In one dish, place the flour.
   - In the second dish, place the beaten eggs.
   - In the third dish, mix together the panko breadcrumbs, salt, pepper, and garlic powder.

3. Working in batches, dredge the chicken pieces in the flour, dip them in the egg, and then coat them in the seasoned panko breadcrumbs, pressing gently to help the crumbs adhere.

4. Arrange the breaded chicken nuggets in a single layer on the prepared baking sheet. Spray the tops of the nuggets lightly with cooking spray.

5. Bake for 12-15 minutes, flipping the nuggets halfway through, until the chicken is cooked through and the breading is golden brown and crispy.

6. Serve the baked chicken nuggets warm, with your favorite dipping sauces like ranch, honey mustard, or barbecue sauce.

Tips:
- For extra crispiness, you can also broil the nuggets for 1-2 minutes after baking.
- Try different seasoning blends in the breadcrumbs, like Italian herbs or Cajun spices.
- Encourage teens to get involved in the breading process for a fun hands-on activity.

Did you have fun cooking this dish?

 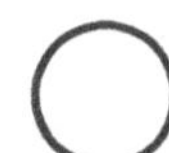 ◯    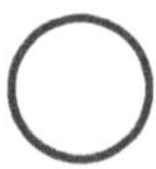 ◯

How would you rate this dish?

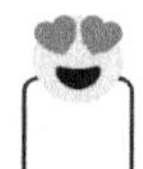 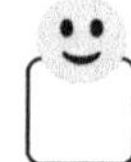 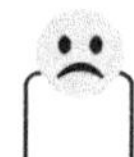 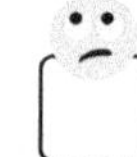 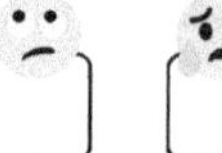

Welcome to ***"The Complete Cookbook for Young Teens: Empower Young Chefs with Nutritious Meals and Tasty Snacks They Can Make Themselves."*** This cookbook is designed specifically for young aspiring chefs who are eager to explore the world of cooking and create delicious meals and snacks right in their own kitchen.

Cooking is not just a valuable life skill; it's a creative and empowering activity that allows you to express yourself while nourishing your body. Whether you're brand new to the kitchen or have some experience, this book is here to guide you through every step of the culinary journey.

Why This Cookbook? *Cooking as a young teen can be incredibly rewarding for several reasons:*

- ***Independence:*** Learn how to prepare meals and snacks on your own, gaining confidence and independence in the kitchen.

- ***Nutrition:*** Discover the importance of balanced meals and snacks that provide energy and support your growing body.

- ***Creativity:*** Explore new flavors, ingredients, and techniques to unleash your creativity and develop your own unique cooking style.

- ***Family and Friends:*** Impress your family and friends with delicious dishes you've prepared yourself, creating memorable moments around the table.

What You'll Find Inside:
- ***Over 100 Recipes:*** From quick and easy snacks to hearty meals, each recipe is designed with young chefs in mind, featuring clear instructions and simple ingredients.

- ***Nutritional Tips:*** Learn about the nutritional benefits of different ingredients and how to make healthy choices without sacrificing taste.

- ***Kitchen Basics:*** Master essential cooking techniques, from chopping vegetables to using kitchen appliances safely and effectively.

- ***Fun and Engaging:*** Enjoy cooking with recipes that are not only nutritious but also fun to make, ensuring that you have a great time in the kitchen.

Get Ready to Cook!

Whether you're cooking for yourself, family, or friends, "The Complete Cookbook for Young Teens" is your go-to guide for delicious and nutritious meals and snacks. Let this book be your companion as you embark on a culinary adventure, discovering new flavors and mastering essential cooking skills along the way. Get ready to unleash your inner chef, experiment with different recipes, and create meals that will make you proud. Cooking is a journey of exploration and enjoyment, and with this cookbook, you have everything you need to succeed.

Let's start cooking and have fun making meals that not only taste great but also nourish your body and mind!

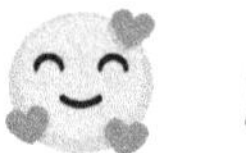 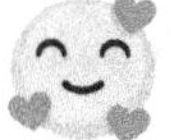 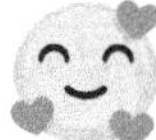 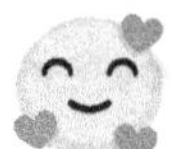 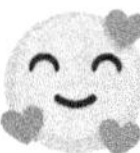 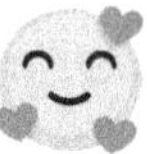 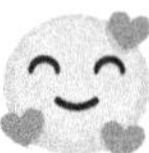 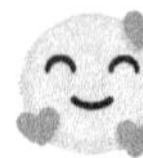  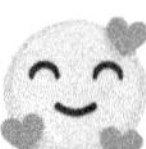

1. Cheeseburgers

Let's do that and fill in the time here  Prep Time :   Cook Time :   Servings :

Write 5 friends with whom you want to share this dish

....
....
....
....

Is this dish easy or difficult for you to make?

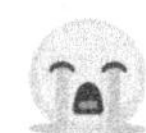 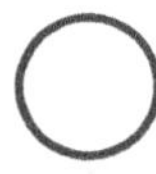 ◯   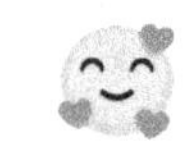 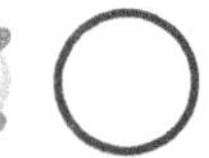 ◯

INGREDIENTS

- 1 lb ground beef
- 4 hamburger buns, split
- 4 slices cheddar cheese
- Lettuce, tomato, onion (optional toppings)
- Condiments like ketchup, mustard, mayo (optional)

1. Form the ground beef into 4 equal-sized patties, about 4-5 inches wide and 1/2 inch thick. Season the patties with salt and pepper.

2. Preheat a grill or grill pan over medium-high heat. Cook the patties for 3-4 minutes per side, until cooked through and the internal temperature reaches 160°F.

3. During the last minute of cooking, top each patty with a slice of cheddar cheese to melt.

4. Place the cheeseburger patties on the buns. Top with desired toppings like lettuce, tomato, onion, ketchup, mustard, mayo, etc.

5. Serve the cheeseburgers immediately while the cheese is melted.

Tips:
- For extra flavor, you can mix in seasonings like garlic powder, onion powder, or Worcestershire sauce into the ground beef before forming the patties.
- Toast the buns lightly before assembling the burgers.
- Consider adding bacon, pickles, or other favorite toppings.

Enjoy your homemade cheeseburgers!

Did you have fun cooking this dish?

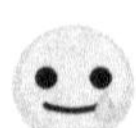 ◯    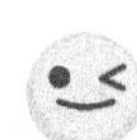 ◯ 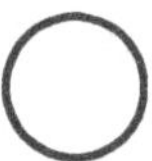

How would you rate this dish?

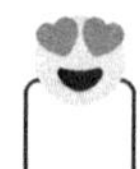 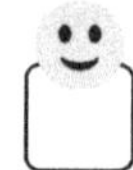  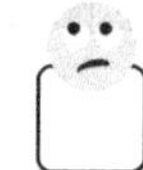 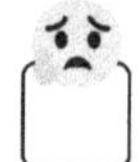

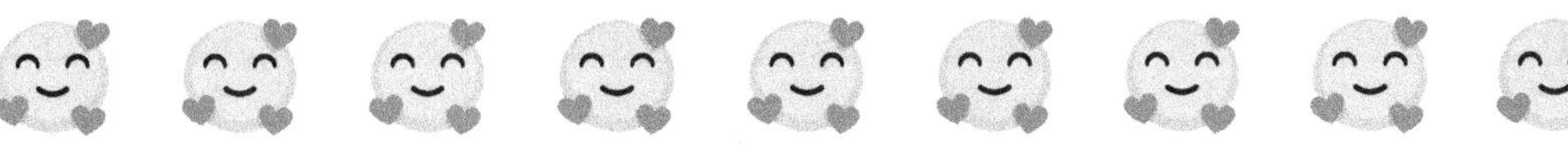

4. French fries

 Prep Time : 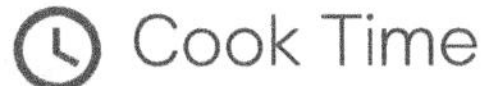 Cook Time : 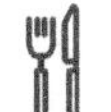 Servings :

Write 5 friends with whom you want to share this dish

....
....
....
....
....

INGREDIENTS

- 3 lbs russet potatoes, peeled and cut into 1/4-inch thick fries
- 2 tbsp olive oil or vegetable oil
- 1 tsp salt
- 1/2 tsp black pepper
- Optional seasonings: garlic powder, paprika, chili powder, etc.

Is this dish easy or difficult for you to make?

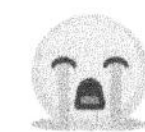 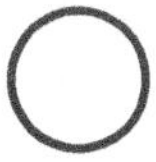 ◯   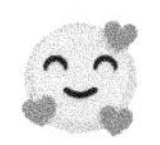  ◯

1. Preheat the oven to 400°F. Line two large baking sheets with parchment paper or silicone baking mats.

2. Place the cut potato fries in a large bowl and cover with cold water to prevent them from browning.

3. Drain the potatoes and pat them very dry with paper towels or a clean kitchen towel. This is important for getting them crispy.

4. In a large bowl, toss the dried potato fries with the oil, salt, and pepper until evenly coated.

5. Spread the fries out in a single layer on the prepared baking sheets, making sure they don't touch each other.

6. Bake for 25-30 minutes, flipping the fries halfway through, until they are golden brown and crispy.

7. Remove the fries from the oven and season with any additional desired seasonings.

8. Serve the crispy baked French fries hot, with ketchup, ranch, or other dipping sauces on the side.

Tips:
- For extra crispiness, soak the cut potatoes in cold water for 30 minutes before baking.
- Try different potato varieties like Yukon Gold or sweet potatoes.
- Encourage teens to experiment with their own seasoning blends.
- Serve the fries alongside burgers, chicken nuggets, or other teen-friendly main dishes.

Did you have fun cooking this dish?

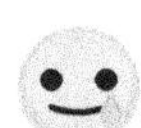 ◯   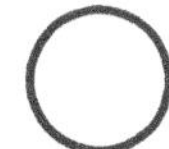 ◯

How would you rate this dish?

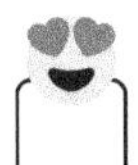 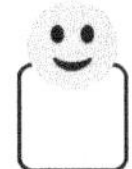  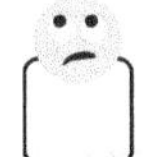 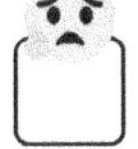

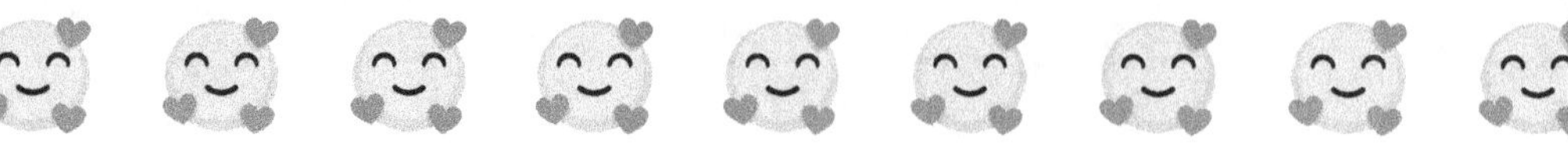

5. Macaroni and cheese

 Prep Time : 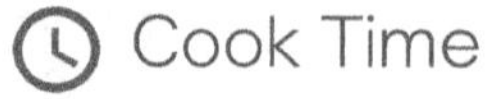 Cook Time : 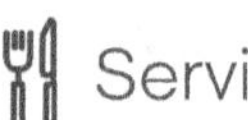 Servings :

Write 5 friends with whom you want to share this dish

....
....
....
....
....

INGREDIENTS

- 8 oz elbow macaroni
- 2 tbsp butter
- 2 tbsp all-purpose flour
- 2 cups milk
- 2 cups shredded cheddar cheese
- 1/2 tsp salt
- 1/4 tsp black pepper

Is this dish easy or difficult for you to make?

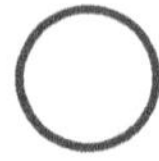 ◯   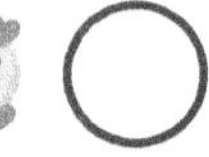 ◯

1. Cook the macaroni according to package directions. Drain and set aside.

2. In a medium saucepan, melt the butter over medium heat. Whisk in the flour and cook for 1 minute, stirring constantly.

3. Gradually whisk in the milk. Bring the mixture to a simmer and cook, stirring frequently, until thickened slightly, about 5 minutes.

4. Remove the sauce from heat and stir in 1 1/2 cups of the shredded cheddar cheese until melted and smooth. Season with salt and pepper.

5. Add the cooked macaroni to the cheese sauce and stir to combine.

6. Transfer the macaroni and cheese to a baking dish and top with the remaining 1/2 cup shredded cheese.

7. Bake at 375°F for 15-20 minutes, until the cheese on top is melted and bubbly.

8. Let stand for 5 minutes before serving.

This homemade mac and cheese is super easy to make and has a creamy, cheesy sauce that teens are sure to love. You can also try adding in some cooked bacon, diced ham, or steamed broccoli for extra flavor and nutrition. Enjoy!

Did you have fun cooking this dish?

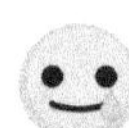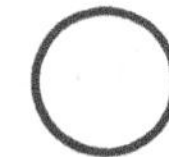 ◯   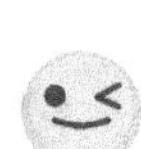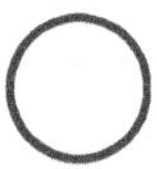 ◯

How would you rate this dish?

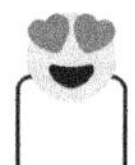  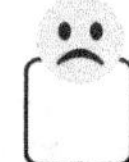 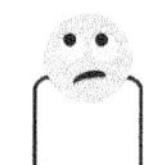 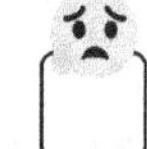

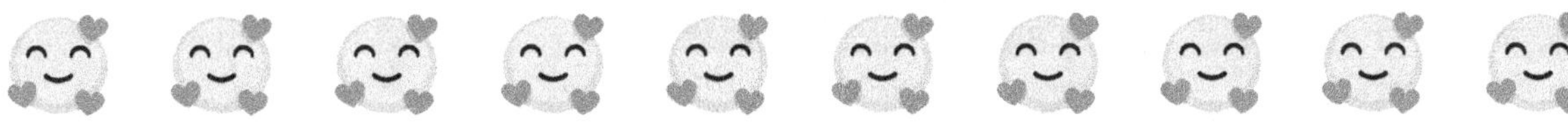

6. Spaghetti and meatballs

 Prep Time :

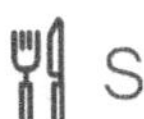 Cook Time :

Servings :

Write 5 friends with whom you want to share this dish

....

....

....

....

....

Is this dish easy or difficult for you to make?

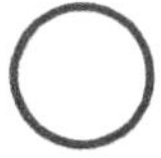 ◯   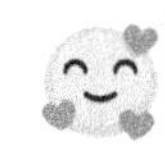 ◯

INGREDIENTS

Meatballs:
- 1 lb ground beef
- 1/2 cup breadcrumbs
- 1/4 cup grated Parmesan cheese
- 1 egg, beaten
- 2 cloves garlic, minced
- 1 tsp dried oregano
- 1/2 tsp salt
- 1/4 tsp black pepper

Spaghetti and Sauce:
- 12 oz spaghetti pasta
- 1 jar (24 oz) marinara sauce
- 2 tbsp olive oil
- 2 cloves garlic, minced
- 1/4 cup fresh basil leaves, chopped (optional)

Meatballs:
1. In a large bowl, combine all the meatball ingredients and mix well until fully incorporated.
2. Roll the mixture into 1-inch meatballs and place them on a baking sheet.
3. Bake the meatballs at 400°F for 15-18 minutes, until cooked through.

Spaghetti and Sauce:
1. Bring a large pot of salted water to a boil. Cook the spaghetti according to package instructions until al dente. Drain and set aside.
2. In a large skillet, heat the olive oil over medium heat. Add the minced garlic and cook for 1 minute until fragrant.
3. Pour in the marinara sauce and add the cooked meatballs. Simmer for 5-10 minutes to allow the flavors to meld.
4. Add the cooked spaghetti to the sauce and toss to coat.
5. Serve the spaghetti and meatballs warm, garnished with fresh chopped basil if desired.

Tips:
- For extra flavor, add Italian seasoning or red pepper flakes to the meatball mixture.
- Use a combination of ground beef and ground pork for the meatballs.
- Encourage teens to get involved in rolling the meatballs.
- Serve with a side salad or garlic bread for a complete meal.

This classic spaghetti and meatballs dish is a crowd-pleasing favorite that young teens are sure to enjoy.

Did you have fun cooking this dish?

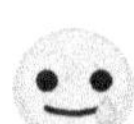 ◯    ◯

How would you rate this dish?

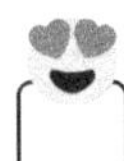   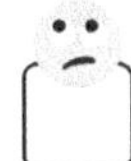 

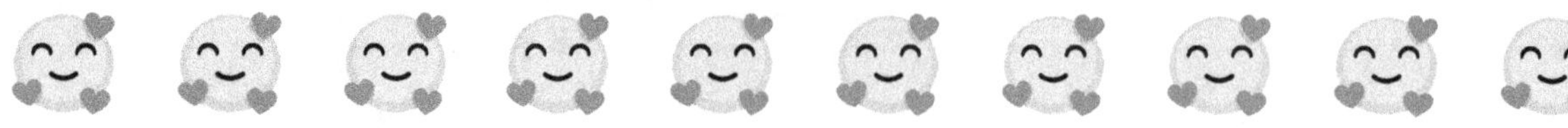

7. Tacos

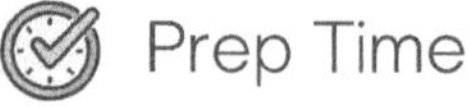 Prep Time :   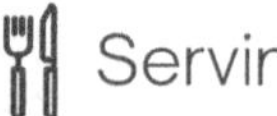 Cook Time :   Servings :

Write 5 friends with whom you want to share this dish

INGREDIENTS

- 1 lb ground beef or ground turkey
- 1 packet taco seasoning
- 1/2 cup water
- 8-10 taco shells or soft tortillas
- Shredded lettuce
- Diced tomatoes
- Shredded cheese (cheddar or Mexican blend)
- Sour cream (optional)
- Salsa (optional)

Did you have fun cooking this dish?

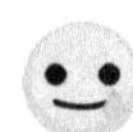 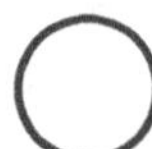    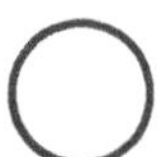

How would you rate this dish?

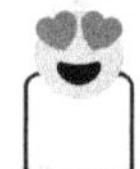 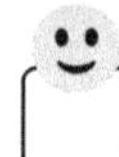 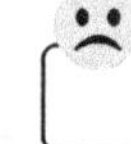 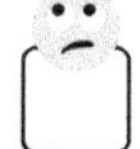 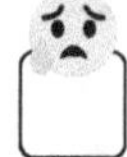

Is this dish easy or difficult for you to make?

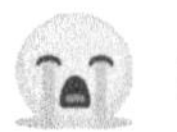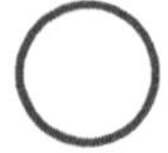   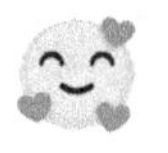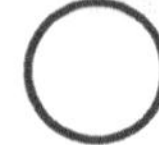

1. In a skillet over medium heat, cook the ground beef or turkey until browned and crumbled, 5-7 minutes. Drain any excess fat.

2. Add the taco seasoning and water to the skillet. Stir to combine and let simmer for 5 minutes, until the sauce has thickened.

3. Warm the taco shells or tortillas according to package instructions.

4. To assemble the tacos, layer the seasoned meat, shredded lettuce, diced tomatoes, and shredded cheese into the taco shells or tortillas.

5. Top with a dollop of sour cream and/or salsa if desired.

6. Serve immediately and enjoy!

You can customize the toppings to your liking, such as adding diced onions, jalapeños, guacamole, or black olives. This is a classic and easy taco recipe that's perfect for a quick weeknight meal.

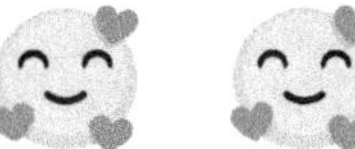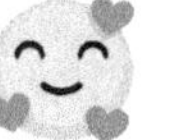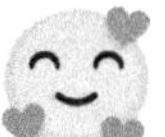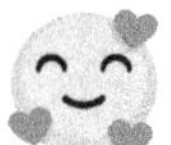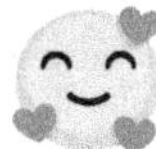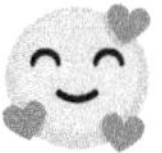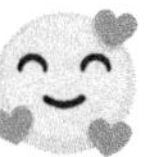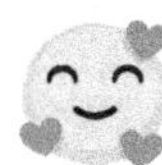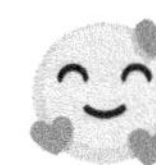

8. Nachos

Let's do that and fill in the time here

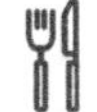 Prep Time :

Cook Time :

Servings :

Write 5 friends with whom you want to share this dish

....

....

....

....

....

Is this dish easy or difficult for you to make?

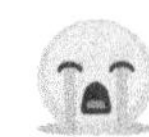 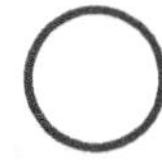 ◯   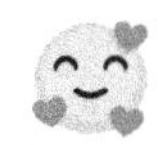 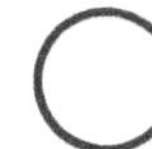 ◯

INGREDIENTS

- 1 bag of tortilla chips
- 1 lb ground beef or turkey
- 1 packet taco seasoning
- 1/2 cup water
- 1 (15 oz) can black beans, drained and rinsed
- 2 cups shredded cheddar or Mexican blend cheese
- Diced tomatoes
- Sliced black olives (optional)
- Sour cream (optional)
- Salsa (optional)

1. Preheat your oven to 375°F.

2. In a skillet over medium heat, cook the ground beef or turkey until browned and crumbled, about 5-7 minutes. Drain any excess fat.

3. Add the taco seasoning and water to the skillet. Stir to combine and let simmer for 5 minutes, until the sauce has thickened.

4. Spread the tortilla chips out in a single layer on a large baking sheet or oven-safe platter.

5. Top the chips evenly with the cooked seasoned meat, black beans, and shredded cheese.

6. Bake for 10-15 minutes, until the cheese is melted and bubbly.

7. Remove the nachos from the oven and top with diced tomatoes, sliced black olives, sour cream, and/or salsa, if desired.

8. Serve the nachos immediately while hot and enjoy!

This nachos recipe is super easy to make and perfect for a quick snack or light meal. The combination of seasoned ground meat, beans, melty cheese, and fresh toppings is sure to be a hit with young teens. You can also let them customize their own nachos with their favorite toppings.

Did you have fun cooking this dish?

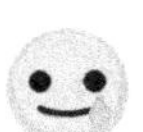 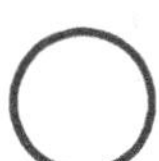 ◯    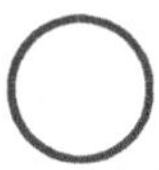 ◯

How would you rate this dish?

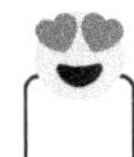 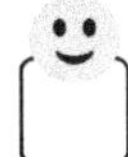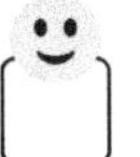 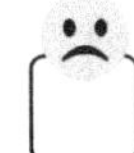 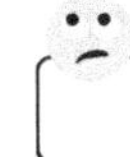 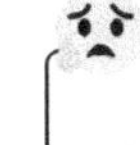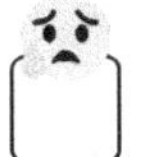

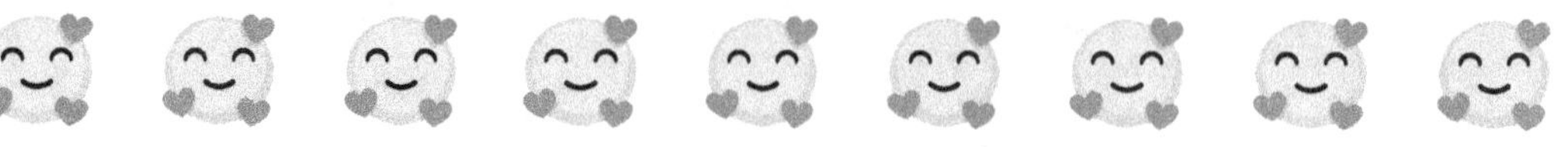

9. Quesadillas

 Prep Time : 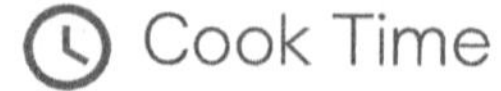 Cook Time :  Servings :

Is this dish easy or difficult for you to make?

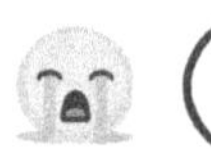 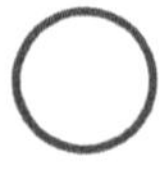 ◯   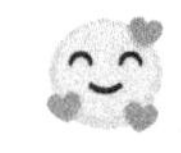 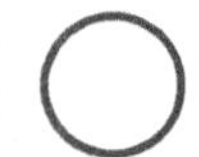 ◯

Write 5 friends with whom you want to share this dish

INGREDIENTS

- 8 medium-sized flour tortillas
- 2 cups shredded cheddar or Mexican blend cheese
- 1 lb boneless, skinless chicken breasts (or 1 lb ground beef/turkey)
- 1 packet taco seasoning
- 1/2 cup water
- Diced tomatoes (optional)
- Sliced black olives (optional)
- Sour cream (optional)
- Salsa (optional)

Did you have fun cooking this dish?

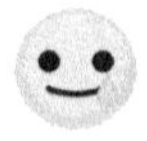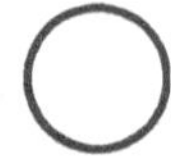 ◯   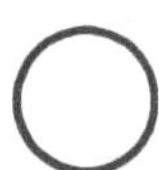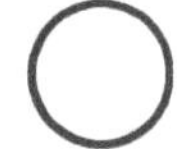 ◯

How would you rate this dish?

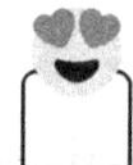 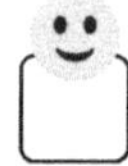  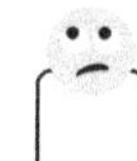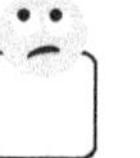 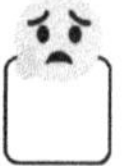

1. If using chicken, cook it in a skillet over medium heat until no longer pink, about 6-8 minutes per side. Shred or dice the cooked chicken.

2. If using ground beef or turkey, cook it in a skillet over medium heat until browned and crumbled, about 5-7 minutes. Drain any excess fat.

3. Add the taco seasoning and water to the cooked meat. Stir to combine and let simmer for 5 minutes, until the sauce has thickened.

4. Lay 4 of the tortillas out on a flat surface. Evenly distribute the shredded cheese and cooked seasoned meat over the tortillas.

5. Top each quesadilla with another tortilla to create 4 complete quesadillas.

6. Heat a large skillet or griddle over medium heat. Cook the quesadillas one or two at a time, for 2-3 minutes per side, until the tortillas are lightly browned and the cheese is melted.

7. Cut the quesadillas into wedges and serve with diced tomatoes, sliced black olives, sour cream, and/or salsa on the side.

This quesadilla recipe is super easy to make and perfect for a quick lunch or dinner. The combination of the warm, melty cheese and seasoned meat is sure to be a hit with young teens. You can also let them customize their own quesadillas with their favorite toppings.

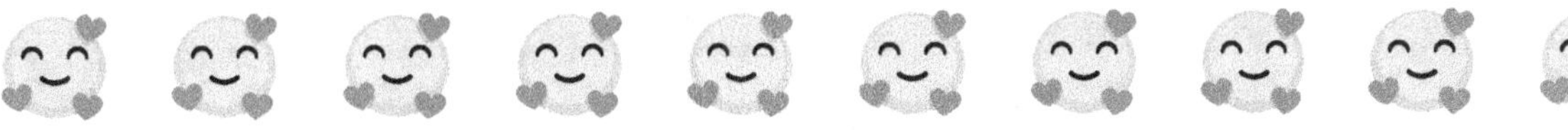

10. Grilled cheese sandwiches

 Prep Time : 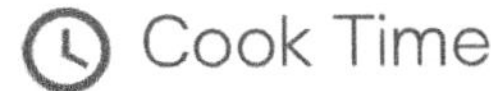 Cook Time :  Servings :

Write 5 friends with whom you want to share this dish
....
....
....
....
....

INGREDIENTS

- 8 slices of bread (white, sourdough, or whole wheat)
- 8 slices of cheddar, American, or Swiss cheese
- 4 tbsp butter, softened

Is this dish easy or difficult for you to make?

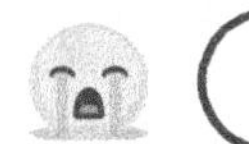 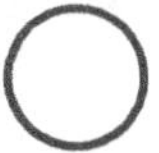 ◯  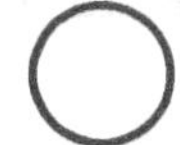 ◯

1. Preheat a skillet or griddle over medium heat.

2. Lay 4 slices of bread out on a flat surface. Top each slice with 2 slices of cheese.

3. Place the remaining 4 slices of bread on top to create 4 complete sandwiches.

4. Spread the softened butter evenly on the outside of each sandwich.

5. Place the sandwiches in the preheated skillet or griddle. Cook for 2-3 minutes per side, until the bread is golden brown and the cheese is melted.

6. Carefully flip the sandwiches and cook the other side for another 2-3 minutes.

7. Remove the grilled cheese sandwiches from the heat and let cool for 1-2 minutes before serving.

Variations:

- Add a slice of tomato or bacon for extra flavor.
- Use different types of cheese, like cheddar and Swiss.
- Spread a thin layer of mayonnaise on the bread instead of butter.
- Sprinkle a little garlic powder or Italian seasoning on the bread before grilling.

This classic grilled cheese recipe is super easy for teens to make and customize to their liking. Serve it with a side of tomato soup or a fresh salad for a complete and satisfying meal. Enjoy!

Did you have fun cooking this dish?

 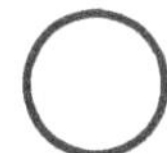 ◯  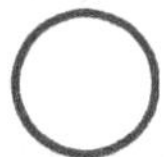 ◯

How would you rate this dish?

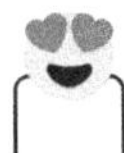 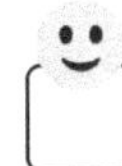 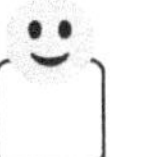  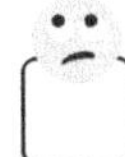 

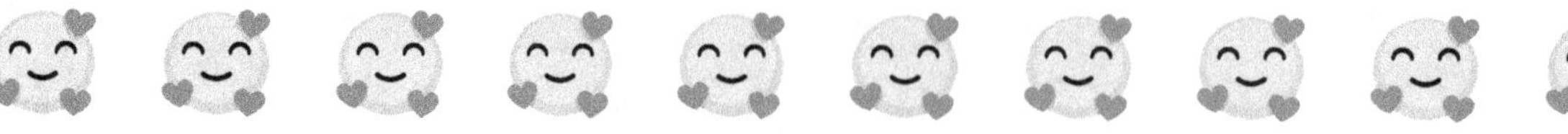

11. Hot dogs

 Prep Time : 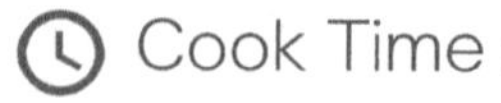 Cook Time : 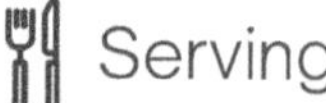 Servings :

Is this dish easy or difficult for you to make?

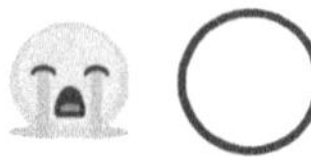 ◯   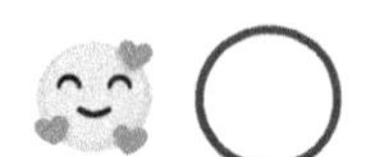 ◯

Write 5 friends with whom you want to share this dish

....
....
....
....
....

INGREDIENTS

- 8 hot dogs
- 8 hot dog buns
- Condiments (such as ketchup, mustard, relish, onions, etc.)

1. Bring a large pot of water to a boil over high heat. Carefully add the hot dogs and let them cook for 5-7 minutes, until heated through.

2. Alternatively, you can grill the hot dogs over medium-high heat for 5-7 minutes, turning occasionally, until heated through and lightly charred. Place each hot dog in a hot dog bun.

3. Allow teens to customize their hot dogs with their favorite condiments, such as:
   - Ketchup - Mustard
   - Relish   - Diced onions
   - Sauerkraut   - Chili
   - Cheese

5. Serve the hot dogs immediately while hot.

Variations:

- For chili cheese dogs, top the hot dogs with warm chili and shredded cheddar cheese.
- For corn dogs, dip the hot dogs in a cornmeal batter before frying or baking.
- For Hawaiian dogs, top the hot dogs with grilled pineapple slices and teriyaki sauce.
- For veggie dogs, use plant-based hot dog alternatives.

Hot dogs are a classic and easy-to-make meal that most teens enjoy. This simple recipe allows them to customize their hot dogs with their favorite toppings, making it a fun and interactive meal. Serve with some baked beans, potato salad, or a fresh veggie side for a complete and satisfying meal.

Did you have fun cooking this dish?

 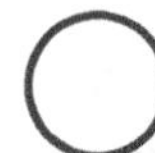 ◯     ◯

How would you rate this dish?

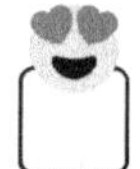 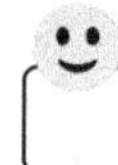  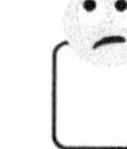 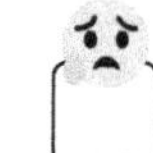

 *Let's do that and fill in the time here*

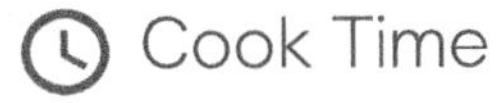 Prep Time :

 Cook Time :

Servings :

Write 5 friends with whom you want to share this dish

....

....

....

....

INGREDIENTS

- 1 lb boneless, skinless chicken breasts, cut into strips
- 1 cup all-purpose flour
- 1 tsp salt
- 1/2 tsp black pepper
- 2 eggs, beaten
- 1 cup panko breadcrumbs
- 1/2 cup grated Parmesan cheese
- 1 tsp garlic powder
- 1 tsp paprika
- Vegetable oil for frying

Did you have fun cooking this dish?

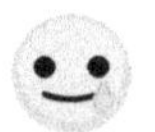 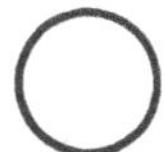  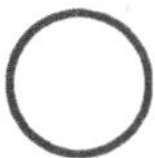

How would you rate this dish?

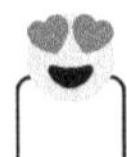 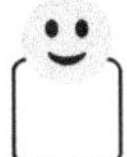 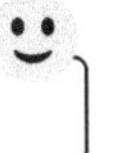 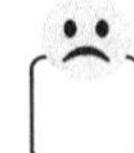 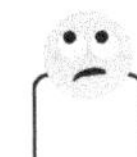 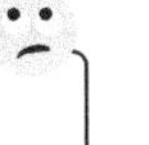 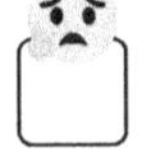

Is this dish easy or difficult for you to make?

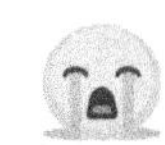 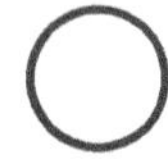 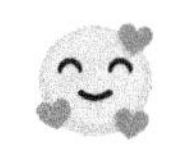 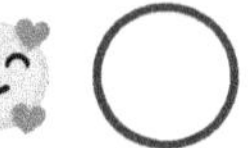

1. Set up a breading station with three shallow dishes:
   - In the first dish, place the flour, salt, and pepper. Mix to combine.
   - In the second dish, place the beaten eggs.
   - In the third dish, mix together the panko, Parmesan, garlic powder, and paprika.

2. Dredge the chicken strips in the flour mixture, dip them in the egg, and then coat them in the panko mixture, pressing gently to adhere.

3. In a large skillet, heat about 1/2 inch of vegetable oil over medium-high heat.

4. Working in batches, fry the breaded chicken tenders for 2-3 minutes per side, until golden brown and cooked through.

5. Transfer the fried chicken tenders to a paper towel-lined plate to drain any excess oil. Serve the chicken tenders warm, with your favorite dipping sauces like ranch, honey mustard, or barbecue sauce.

Tips:
- For extra crispy tenders, let the breaded chicken sit for 10-15 minutes before frying.
- Bake the tenders at 400°F for 15-20 minutes instead of frying for a healthier option.
- Try different seasoning blends in the breading, like Cajun or lemon pepper.

These homemade chicken tenders are sure to be a hit with young teens. They're crispy on the outside and juicy on the inside, making them a delicious and satisfying meal or snack. Enjoy!

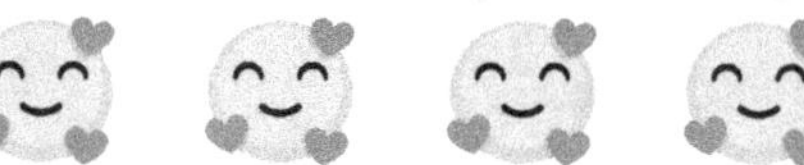

13. Mozzarella sticks

 Prep Time :   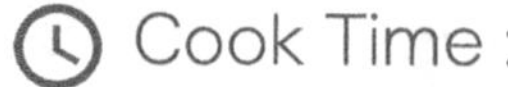  Cook Time :   Servings :

Let's do that and fill in the time here

Write 5 friends with whom you want to share this dish

....
....
....
....
....

Is this dish easy or difficult for you to make?

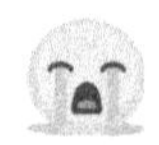 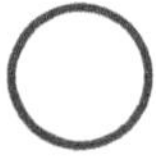 ◯   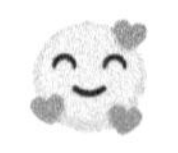 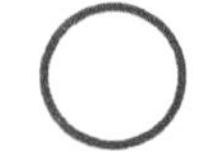 ◯

INGREDIENTS

- 8 oz block of mozzarella cheese, cut into 1/2-inch thick sticks
- 1 cup all-purpose flour
- 2 eggs, beaten
- 1 cup panko breadcrumbs
- 1/2 cup grated Parmesan cheese
- 1 tsp garlic powder
- 1 tsp dried oregano
- 1/2 tsp salt
- Vegetable oil for frying
- Marinara sauce or ranch dressing for dipping

1. Set up a breading station with three shallow dishes:
   - In the first dish, place the flour.
   - In the second dish, place the beaten eggs.
   - In the third dish, mix together the panko, Parmesan, garlic powder, oregano, and salt.

2. Dredge the mozzarella sticks in the flour, dip them in the egg, and then coat them in the panko mixture, pressing gently to adhere.

3. In a large skillet, heat about 1/2 inch of vegetable oil over medium-high heat.

4. Working in batches, fry the breaded mozzarella sticks for 1-2 minutes per side, until golden brown.

5. Transfer the fried mozzarella sticks to a paper towel-lined plate to drain any excess oil.

6. Serve the mozzarella sticks warm, with marinara sauce or ranch dressing for dipping.

Tips:
- For extra crispy mozzarella sticks, let the breaded sticks sit in the refrigerator for 30 minutes before frying.
- Bake the mozzarella sticks at 400°F for 10-12 minutes instead of frying for a healthier option.
- Try different seasoning blends in the breading, like Italian seasoning or Cajun spice.

These homemade mozzarella sticks are sure to be a hit with young teens. They're crispy on the outside and gooey on the inside, making them a delicious and satisfying snack or appetizer. Enjoy!

Did you have fun cooking this dish?

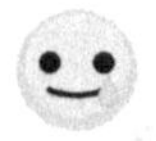 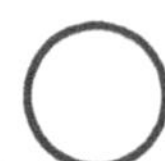 ◯    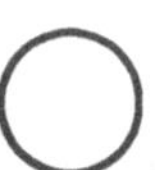 ◯

How would you rate this dish?

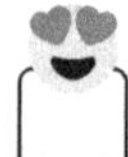 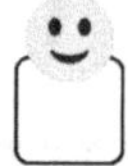 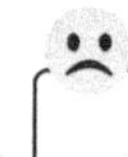 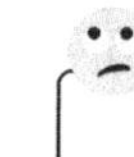 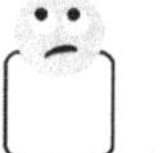 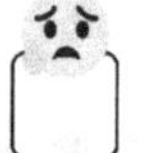

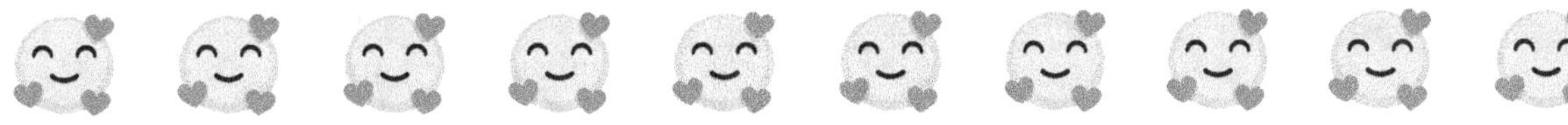

14. Onion rings

 Prep Time : 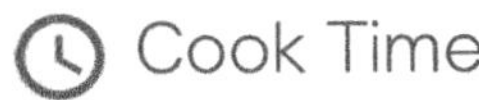 Cook Time : 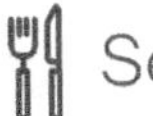 Servings :

Write 5 friends with whom you want to share this dish

....
....
....
....
....

INGREDIENTS

- 2 large onions, sliced into 1/2-inch thick rings
- 1 cup all-purpose flour
- 1 tsp salt
- 1/2 tsp black pepper
- 2 eggs, beaten
- 1 cup panko breadcrumbs
- Vegetable oil for frying

Is this dish easy or difficult for you to make?

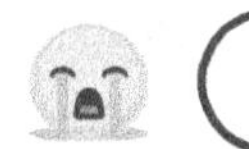 ◯   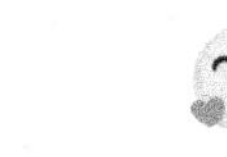 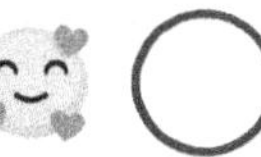 ◯

1. Separate the onion slices into individual rings.

2. In a shallow dish, mix together the flour, salt, and black pepper.

3. In a second shallow dish, place the beaten eggs.

4. In a third shallow dish, place the panko breadcrumbs.

5. Working in batches, dredge the onion rings in the flour mixture, dip them in the beaten eggs, and then coat them in the panko breadcrumbs, pressing gently to adhere.

6. In a large skillet or Dutch oven, heat about 1-2 inches of vegetable oil over medium-high heat to 350°F.

7. Carefully add the breaded onion rings to the hot oil and fry for 2-3 minutes per side, until golden brown and crispy.

8. Transfer the fried onion rings to a paper towel-lined plate to drain any excess oil.

9. Serve the onion rings warm, with your favorite dipping sauces like ranch, barbecue, or honey mustard.

Tips:
- For extra crispy onion rings, let the breaded rings sit in the refrigerator for 30 minutes before frying.
- Bake the onion rings at 400°F for 15-20 minutes instead of frying for a healthier option.
- Try different seasoning blends in the breading, like Cajun spice or garlic powder.

Did you have fun cooking this dish?

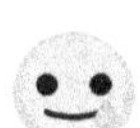 ◯   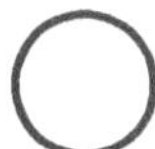 ◯

How would you rate this dish?

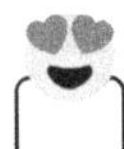 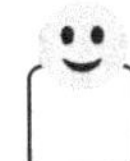   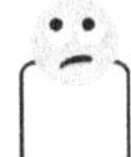 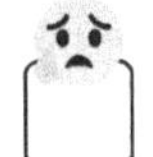

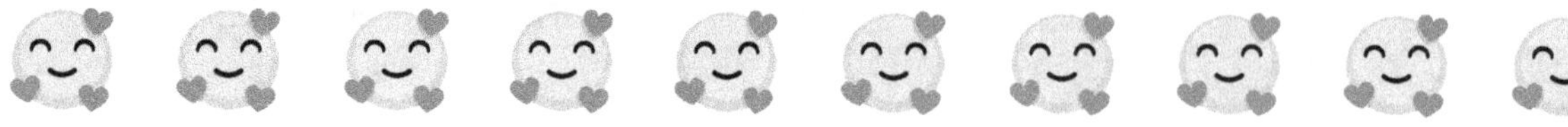

15. Potato skins

 Prep Time :   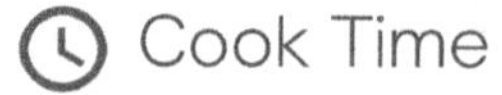 Cook Time :    Servings :

Write 5 friends with whom you want to share this dish

Is this dish easy or difficult for you to make?
◯   ◯

INGREDIENTS

- 4 medium russet potatoes
- 2 tbsp olive oil
- 1 tsp salt
- 1/2 tsp black pepper
- 1 cup shredded cheddar cheese
- 4 slices bacon, cooked and crumbled
- 2 green onions, sliced
- Sour cream for serving (optional)

1. Preheat your oven to 400°F.

2. Wash the potatoes and prick them several times with a fork. Bake the potatoes directly on the oven rack for 50-60 minutes, until tender when pierced with a fork.

3. Let the potatoes cool for 10 minutes, then cut them in half lengthwise. Scoop out the insides, leaving about 1/4 inch of potato flesh attached to the skin.

4. Brush the potato skins with olive oil and season with salt and pepper.

5. Place the potato skins, skin-side up, on a baking sheet. Bake for 10 minutes to crisp up the skins.

6. Remove the potato skins from the oven and flip them over. Top each skin with shredded cheddar cheese and crumbled bacon.

7. Return the potato skins to the oven and bake for an additional 5-7 minutes, until the cheese is melted and bubbly.

8. Top the loaded potato skins with sliced green onions. Serve the potato skins warm, with sour cream on the side for dipping, if desired.

Tips:
- For extra crispy skins, broil the potato skins for 2-3 minutes after adding the toppings.
- Try different toppings like diced jalapeños, chili, or chopped chives.
- Bake the potatoes a day in advance to save time.

Did you have fun cooking this dish?

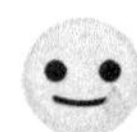 ◯    ◯

How would you rate this dish?

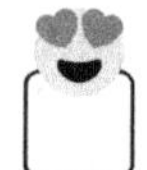 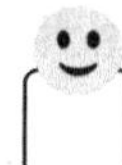 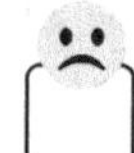 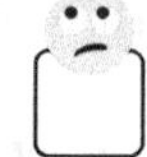 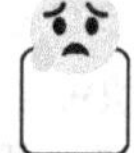

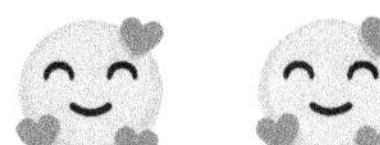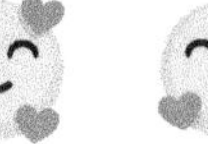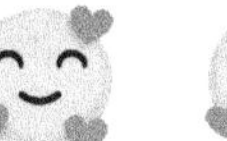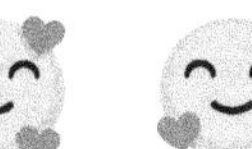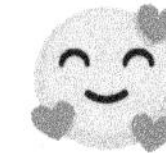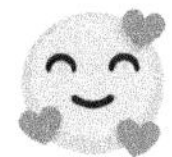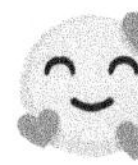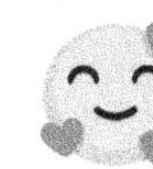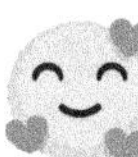

16. Buffalo wings

 Prep Time : 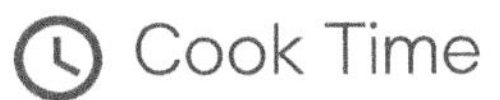 Cook Time : 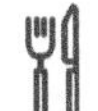 Servings :

Is this dish easy or difficult for you to make?

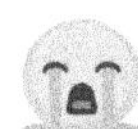 ◯ 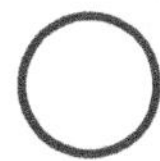   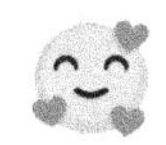 ◯ 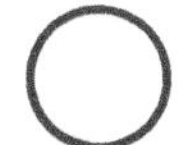

Write 5 friends with whom you want to share this dish

....

....

....

....

....

INGREDIENTS

- 2 lbs chicken wings, drumettes and flats separated
- 1 cup all-purpose flour
- 1 tsp salt
- 1/2 tsp black pepper
- Vegetable oil for frying
- 1/2 cup hot sauce (such as Frank's RedHot)
- 2 tbsp unsalted butter, melted

1. Pat the chicken wings dry with paper towels and place them in a large bowl.

2. In a separate bowl, mix together the flour, salt, and black pepper. Pour the seasoned flour over the wings and toss to coat them evenly.

3. In a large, heavy-bottomed pot or Dutch oven, heat 2-3 inches of vegetable oil to 375°F.

4. Working in batches, carefully add the coated chicken wings to the hot oil and fry for 12-15 minutes, turning occasionally, until golden brown and crispy.

5. Transfer the fried wings to a paper towel-lined plate to drain any excess oil.

6. In a large bowl, whisk together the hot sauce and melted butter.

7. Add the fried wings to the hot sauce mixture and toss to coat them evenly.

8. Serve the buffalo wings immediately, with celery sticks and blue cheese or ranch dressing on the side.

Tips:
- For extra crispy wings, let the coated wings sit in the refrigerator for 30 minutes before frying.
- Bake the wings at 400°F for 40-45 minutes, turning halfway, instead of frying for a healthier option.
- Adjust the amount of hot sauce to your desired level of spiciness.
- Try different sauce flavors, like barbecue or honey garlic.

Did you have fun cooking this dish?

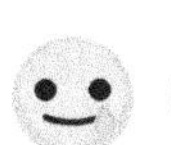 ◯ 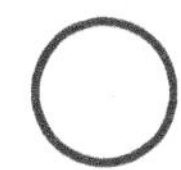    ◯ 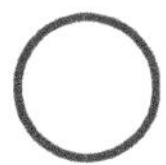

How would you rate this dish?

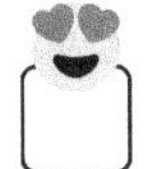 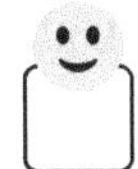 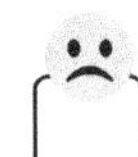 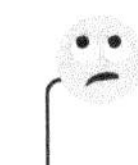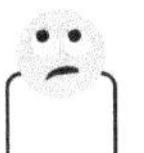 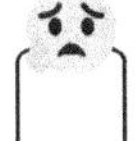

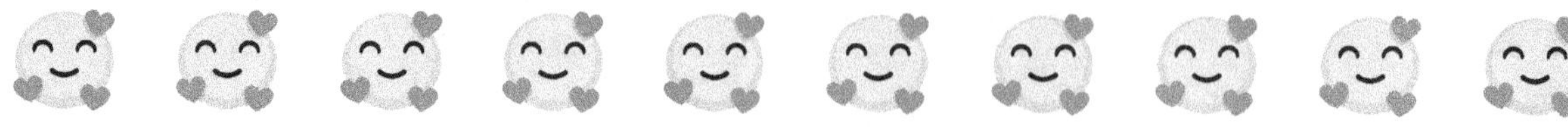

17. Sliders (mini burgers)

 Prep Time : 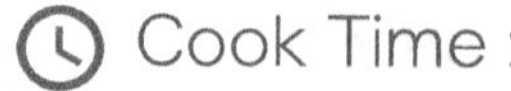 Cook Time :  Servings :

Write 5 friends with whom you want to share this dish

....

....

....

....

....

Is this dish easy or difficult for you to make?

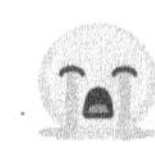 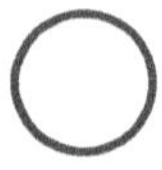 ◯    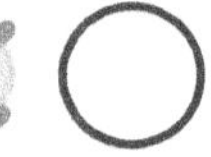 ◯

INGREDIENTS

- 1 lb ground beef
- 1 tsp salt
- 1/2 tsp black pepper
- 12 small dinner rolls or Hawaiian rolls, split in half
- 6 slices cheddar cheese, cut in half
- Toppings (such as lettuce, tomato, onion, pickles)

For the Sauce:
- 1/2 cup mayonnaise
- 2 tbsp ketchup
- 1 tbsp yellow mustard
- 1 tsp dill pickle relish

1. In a large bowl, gently mix together the ground beef, salt, and black pepper until just combined. Avoid overmixing.

2. Divide the beef mixture into 12 equal portions and shape them into small, flat patties, about 2-3 inches in diameter.

3. Preheat a large skillet or griddle over medium-high heat.

4. Cook the slider patties for 2-3 minutes per side, until cooked through.

5. During the last minute of cooking, top each patty with a half slice of cheddar cheese.

6. In a small bowl, mix together the mayonnaise, ketchup, mustard, and pickle relish for the sauce.

7. Place the bottom half of the rolls on a serving platter. Top each with a cheeseburger slider, then add your desired toppings.

8. Spread the sauce on the top half of the rolls and place them on the sliders.

9. Serve the mini cheeseburger sliders immediately, while the cheese is still melted.

Tips:
- For extra flavor, try adding a pinch of garlic powder or onion powder to the beef mixture.
- Experiment with different cheese varieties, such as Swiss or pepper jack.
- Offer a variety of toppings so teens can customize their sliders.

Did you have fun cooking this dish?

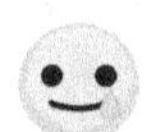 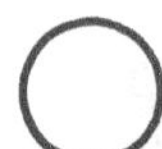 ◯   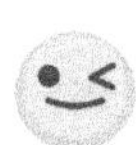 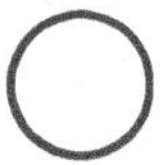 ◯

How would you rate this dish?

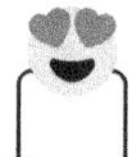 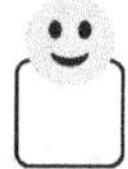 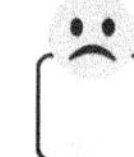 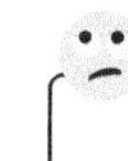 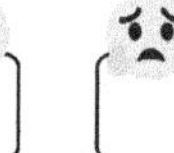

18. Popcorn chicken

Let's do that and fill in the time here 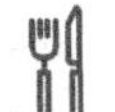 Prep Time :   Cook Time :   Servings :

Is this dish easy or difficult for you to make?

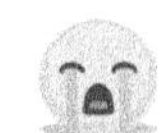 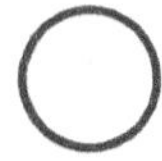 ◯   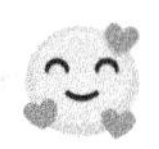 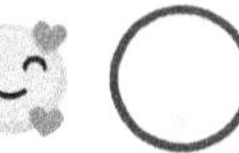 ◯

Write 5 friends with whom you want to share this dish

....

....

....

....

....

INGREDIENTS

- 1 lb boneless, skinless chicken breasts, cut into 1-inch pieces
- 1 cup all-purpose flour
- 1 tsp salt
- 1/2 tsp black pepper
- 2 eggs, beaten
- 1 cup panko breadcrumbs
- Vegetable oil for frying

1. In a shallow dish, mix together the flour, salt, and black pepper.

2. In a second shallow dish, place the beaten eggs.

3. In a third shallow dish, place the panko breadcrumbs.

4. Working in batches, dredge the chicken pieces in the seasoned flour, dip them in the beaten eggs, and then coat them in the panko breadcrumbs, pressing gently to adhere.

5. In a large skillet or Dutch oven, heat about 1-2 inches of vegetable oil over medium-high heat to 350°F.

6. Carefully add the breaded chicken pieces to the hot oil and fry for 2-3 minutes per batch, until golden brown and cooked through.

7. Transfer the fried popcorn chicken to a paper towel-lined plate to drain any excess oil.

8. Serve the popcorn chicken warm, with your favorite dipping sauces like ranch, honey mustard, or barbecue sauce.

Tips:
- For extra crispy popcorn chicken, let the breaded pieces sit in the refrigerator for 30 minutes before frying.
- Bake the popcorn chicken at 400°F for 15-20 minutes instead of frying for a healthier option.
- Try different seasoning blends in the flour, like Cajun spice or lemon pepper.

Did you have fun cooking this dish?

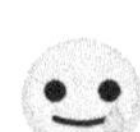 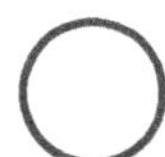 ◯    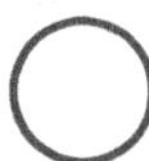 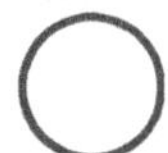 ◯

How would you rate this dish?

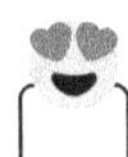 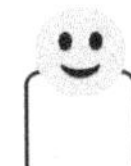  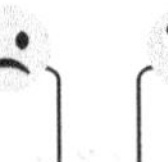 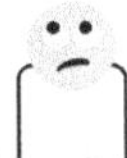 

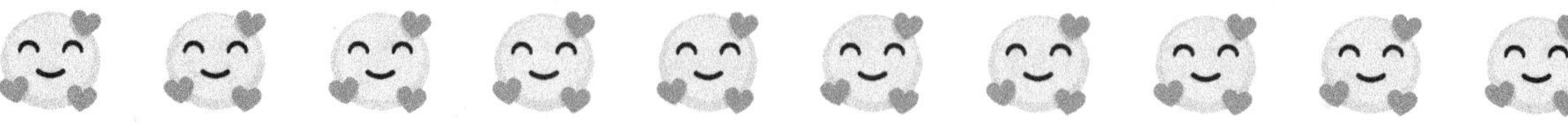

19. Cheese fries

 Prep Time : 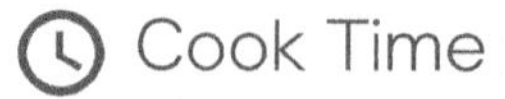 Cook Time : 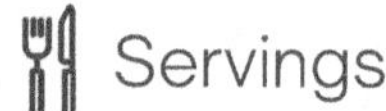 Servings :

Write 5 friends with whom you want to share this dish

....
....
....
....
....

INGREDIENTS

- 3 lbs russet potatoes, cut into 1/4-inch thick fries
- 2 tbsp vegetable oil
- 1 tsp salt
- 1/2 tsp black pepper
- 2 cups shredded cheddar cheese
- 4 slices bacon, cooked and crumbled
- 2 green onions, sliced
- Sour cream for serving (optional)

Is this dish easy or difficult for you to make?

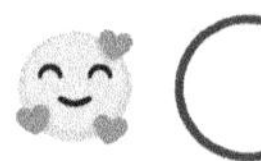 ◯   ◯

1. Preheat your oven to 400°F.

2. Spread the potato fries in a single layer on a large baking sheet. Drizzle with the vegetable oil and season with salt and pepper. Toss to coat.

3. Bake the fries for 25-30 minutes, flipping halfway, until golden brown and crispy.

4. Remove the fries from the oven and top them evenly with the shredded cheddar cheese.

5. Return the fries to the oven and bake for an additional 5-7 minutes, until the cheese is melted and bubbly.

6. Remove the loaded cheese fries from the oven and top them with the crumbled bacon and sliced green onions.

7. Serve the cheese fries warm, with sour cream on the side for dipping, if desired.

Tips:
- For extra crispy fries, soak the cut potatoes in cold water for 30 minutes before drying and baking.
- Try different cheese varieties, such as pepper jack or Monterey Jack.
- Add other toppings like diced jalapeños, chili, or chopped chives.
- Bake the fries a day in advance to save time.

These loaded cheese fries are sure to be a hit with young teens. They're crispy, cheesy, and packed with delicious toppings, making them a perfect snack or side dish. Enjoy!

Did you have fun cooking this dish?

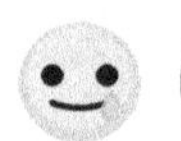 ◯   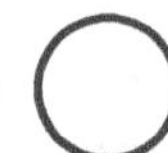 ◯

How would you rate this dish?

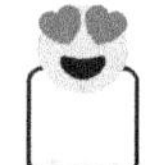 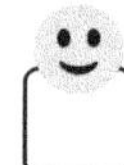  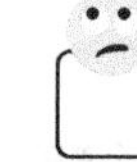 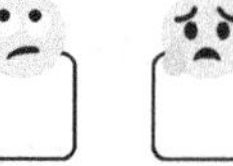

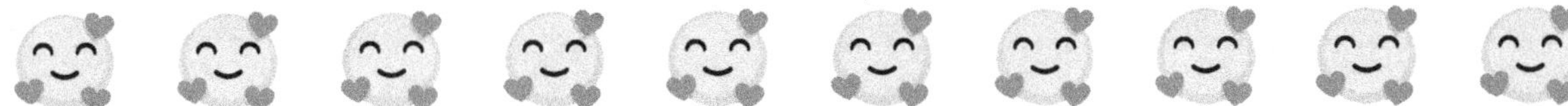

20. Tater tots

 Prep Time :   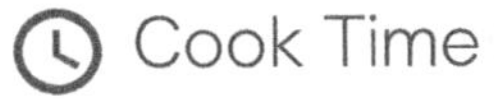  Cook Time :   Servings :

Write 5 friends with whom you want to share this dish

....
....
....
....
....

INGREDIENTS

- 3 lbs russet potatoes, peeled and grated
- 1 tsp salt
- 1/2 tsp black pepper
- 1/4 cup all-purpose flour
- Vegetable oil for frying

Is this dish easy or difficult for you to make?

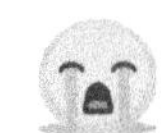 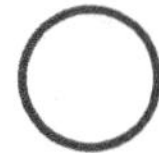 ◯   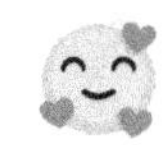 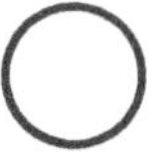 ◯

1. Grate the peeled potatoes using a box grater or the grating attachment of a food processor.

2. Place the grated potatoes in a clean kitchen towel or cheesecloth and squeeze out as much moisture as possible.

3. Transfer the dried potato shreds to a large bowl and season with salt and pepper. Sprinkle the flour over the potatoes and toss to coat.

4. In a large, heavy-bottomed pot or Dutch oven, heat 2-3 inches of vegetable oil to 350°F.

5. Working in batches, carefully drop heaping tablespoons of the potato mixture into the hot oil. Fry for 2-3 minutes, turning occasionally, until golden brown and crispy.

6. Use a slotted spoon to transfer the fried tater tots to a paper towel-lined plate to drain any excess oil.

7. Serve the tater tots warm, with your favorite dipping sauces like ketchup, ranch, or cheese sauce.

Tips:
- For extra crispy tater tots, let the grated potato mixture sit in the refrigerator for 30 minutes before frying.
- Bake the tater tots at 400°F for 20-25 minutes, turning halfway, instead of frying for a healthier option.
- Try adding grated onion, garlic powder, or other seasonings to the potato mixture for extra flavor.

Did you have fun cooking this dish?

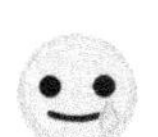 ◯   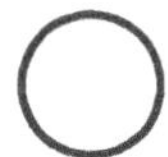 ◯

How would you rate this dish?

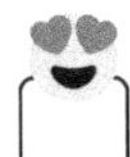 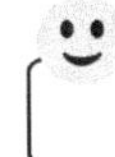 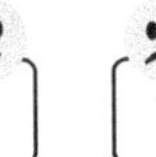 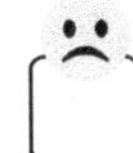 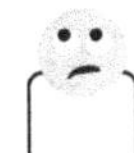 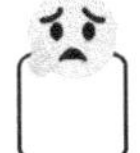

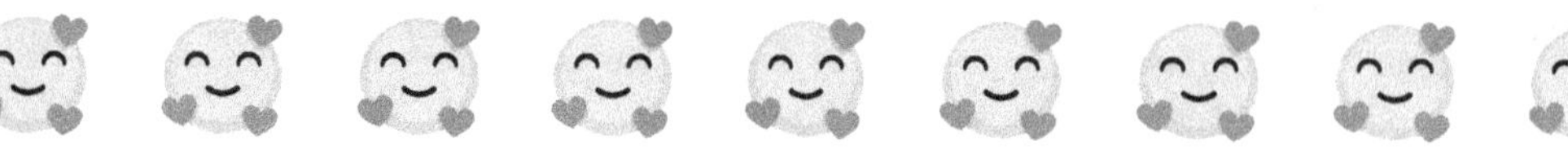

21. Chicken parmesan

 Prep Time : 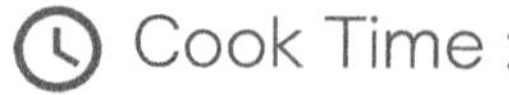 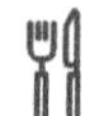 Cook Time : Servings :

Is this dish easy or difficult for you to make?

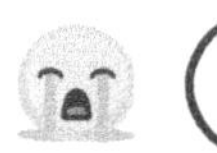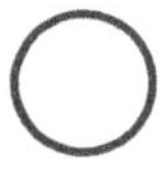 ◯ 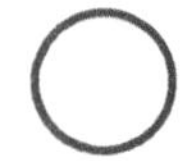 ◯

Write 5 friends with whom you want to share this dish

....

....

....

....

....

INGREDIENTS

- 4 boneless, skinless chicken breasts
- 1 cup all-purpose flour
- 2 eggs, beaten
- 1 cup panko breadcrumbs
- 1 cup grated Parmesan cheese
- 1 tsp dried oregano
- 1/2 tsp garlic powder
- 1/2 tsp salt
- 1/4 tsp black pepper
- 2 cups marinara sauce
- 2 cups shredded mozzarella cheese

1. Preheat your oven to 400°F. Grease a 9x13 inch baking dish.

2. Set up a breading station with three shallow dishes: one with the flour, one with the beaten eggs, and one with the panko breadcrumbs, Parmesan, oregano, garlic powder, salt, and pepper mixed together.

3. Dredge the chicken breasts in the flour, dip them in the egg, and then coat them in the breadcrumb mixture, pressing gently to adhere.

4. Place the breaded chicken in the prepared baking dish.

5. Bake the chicken for 20-25 minutes, until it's cooked through and the breading is golden brown.

6. Remove the chicken from the oven and top each piece with about 1/2 cup of marinara sauce, followed by 1/2 cup of shredded mozzarella cheese.

7. Return the dish to the oven and bake for an additional 10-15 minutes, until the cheese is melted and bubbly.

8. Serve the chicken parmesan immediately, garnished with fresh basil or parsley if desired. Accompany with a side of pasta, garlic bread, or a fresh salad.

This classic chicken parmesan dish is sure to be a hit with young teens. The crispy, breaded chicken topped with melty cheese and marinara sauce is a delicious and satisfying meal. Enjoy!

Did you have fun cooking this dish?

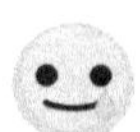 ◯ 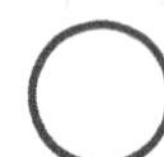 ◯

How would you rate this dish?

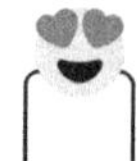 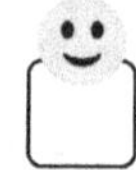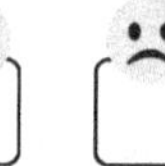  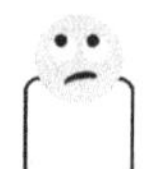 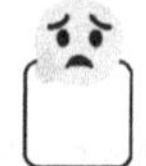

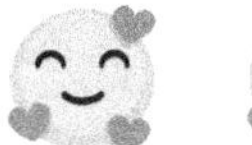 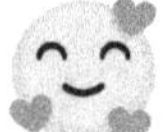 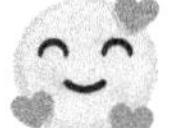 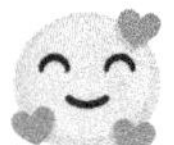 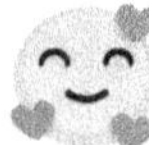 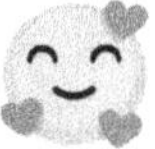 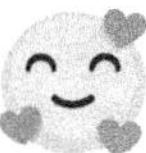 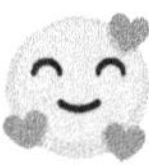 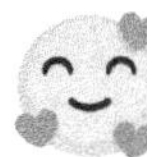 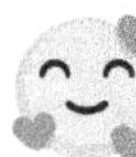

22. Fish and chips

🕐 Prep Time :   🕐 Cook Time :   🍴 Servings :

Write 5 friends with whom you want to share this dish
....
....
....
....
....

Is this dish easy or difficult for you to make?

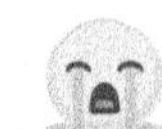 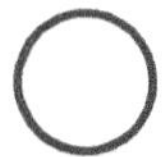 ◯   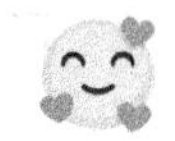 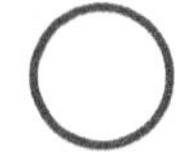 ◯

INGREDIENTS

Fish and Chips

For the Fish:
- 1 lb white fish fillets (such as cod, haddock, or tilapia), cut into 1-inch thick strips
- 1 cup all-purpose flour
- 2 eggs, beaten
- 1 cup panko breadcrumbs
- 1 tsp salt
- 1/2 tsp black pepper
- Vegetable oil for frying

For the Chips (Fries):
- 3 lbs russet potatoes, cut into 1/2-inch thick fries
- 2 tbsp vegetable oil
- 1 tsp salt

For the Fish:
1. Set up a breading station with three shallow dishes: one with the flour, one with the beaten eggs, and one with the panko breadcrumbs mixed with the salt and pepper.
2. Dredge the fish strips in the flour, dip them in the egg, and then coat them in the panko mixture, pressing gently to adhere.
3. In a large, heavy-bottomed pot or Dutch oven, heat 2-3 inches of vegetable oil to 350°F.
4. Working in batches, carefully add the breaded fish strips to the hot oil and fry for 2-3 minutes per side, until golden brown and crispy.
5. Transfer the fried fish to a paper towel-lined plate to drain any excess oil.

For the Chips (Fries):
1. Preheat your oven to 400°F.
2. Spread the cut potato fries in a single layer on a large baking sheet. Drizzle with the vegetable oil and sprinkle with the salt. Toss to coat.
3. Bake the fries for 25-30 minutes, flipping halfway, until golden brown and crispy.

Serve the fried fish and baked fries immediately, with lemon wedges and tartar sauce or malt vinegar on the side.

Tips:
- For extra crispy fish, let the breaded strips sit in the refrigerator for 30 minutes before frying.
- Bake the fries at a higher temperature (425°F) for crispier results.
- Try different types of white fish or even shrimp for variety.

Did you have fun cooking this dish?

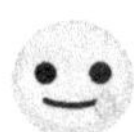 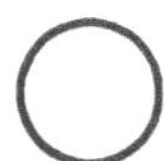 ◯    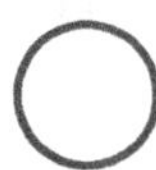 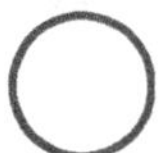 ◯

How would you rate this dish?

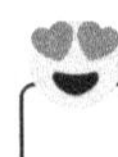 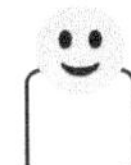  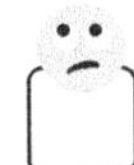 

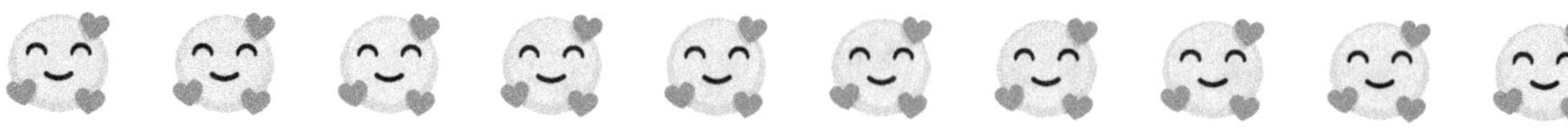

23. Sloppy joes

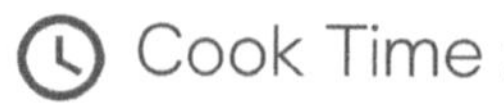 Prep Time :
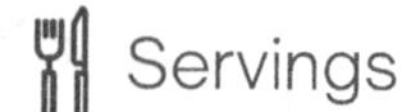 Cook Time :
Servings :

Is this dish easy or difficult for you to make?

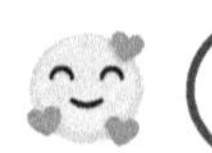

Write 5 friends with whom you want to share this dish

....

....

....

....

INGREDIENTS

- 1 lb ground beef
- 1 onion, diced
- 1 green bell pepper, diced
- 2 cloves garlic, minced
- 1 cup ketchup
- 2 tbsp brown sugar
- 2 tbsp Worcestershire sauce
- 1 tsp mustard powder
- 1/2 tsp chili powder
- 1/4 tsp cayenne pepper (optional)
- Salt and black pepper to taste
- 8 hamburger buns

1. In a large skillet over medium-high heat, cook the ground beef, onion, bell pepper, and garlic until the beef is browned and the vegetables are softened, about 5-7 minutes. Drain any excess fat.

2. Stir in the ketchup, brown sugar, Worcestershire sauce, mustard powder, chili powder, and cayenne pepper (if using). Season with salt and black pepper to taste.

3. Reduce the heat to low and let the sloppy joe mixture simmer for 10-15 minutes, stirring occasionally, until the flavors have melded and the sauce has thickened.

4. Divide the sloppy joe mixture evenly among the hamburger buns.

5. Serve the sloppy joes immediately, with any desired toppings like shredded cheese, pickles, or onions.

Tips:
- For a creamier texture, stir in a tablespoon or two of mayonnaise or sour cream to the sloppy joe mixture.
- Add a splash of apple cider vinegar or hot sauce for a little extra tang and heat.
- Serve the sloppy joes with a side of fries, coleslaw, or a fresh salad for a complete meal.

These classic sloppy joes are sure to be a hit with young teens. The sweet and savory flavors, combined with the messy, handheld nature of the dish, make it a fun and satisfying meal. Enjoy!

Did you have fun cooking this dish?

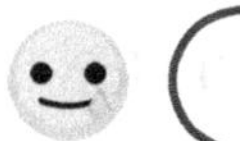 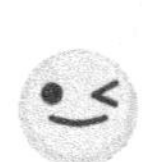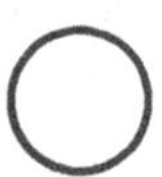

How would you rate this dish?

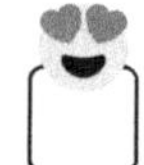 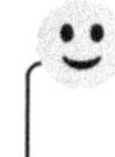  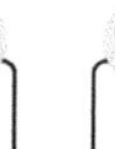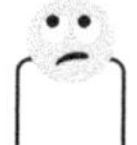 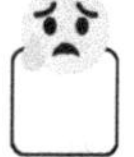

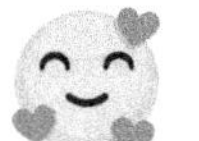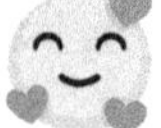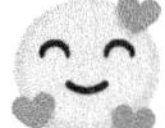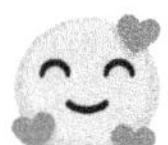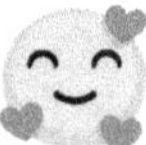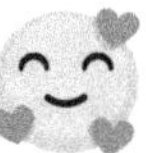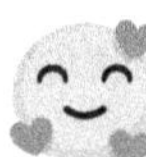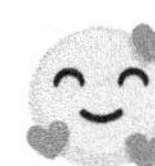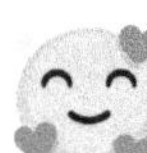

24. Pigs in a blanket

  Prep Time :   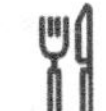 Cook Time :   Servings :

Is this dish easy or difficult for you to make?

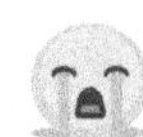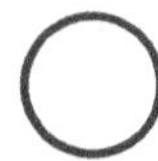 ◯   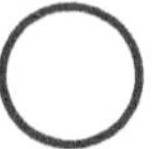 ◯

Write 5 friends with whom you want to share this dish

....

....

....

....

....

INGREDIENTS

- 1 package (8 count) refrigerated crescent roll dough
- 8 hot dogs, cut in half crosswise
- 1 egg, beaten with 1 tbsp water (for egg wash)
- Sesame seeds or poppy seeds (optional)

1. Preheat your oven to 375°F. Line a baking sheet with parchment paper.

2. Unroll the crescent roll dough and separate it into 8 triangles.

3. Place a hot dog half at the wide end of each triangle. Tightly roll the dough around the hot dog, starting at the wide end and ending at the point.

4. Place the wrapped hot dogs seam-side down on the prepared baking sheet.

5. Brush the tops of the pigs in a blanket with the egg wash. Sprinkle with sesame seeds or poppy seeds, if desired.

6. Bake for 12-15 minutes, until the dough is golden brown and flaky.

7. Serve the pigs in a blanket warm, with your favorite dipping sauces like mustard, ketchup, or barbecue sauce.

Tips:
- For extra flavor, try using different types of sausages or hot dogs, such as mini cocktail franks or Italian sausages.
- Experiment with different types of dough, like puff pastry or biscuit dough, instead of crescent rolls.
- Add shredded cheese or chopped bacon to the filling for a delicious twist.

These homemade pigs in a blanket are sure to be a hit with young teens. They're easy to make, portable, and perfect for snacking or serving as an appetizer. Enjoy!

Did you have fun cooking this dish?

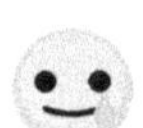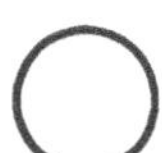 ◯   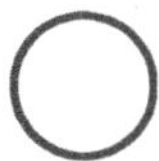 ◯

How would you rate this dish?

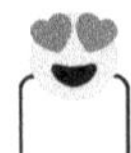 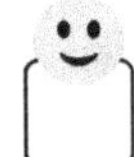 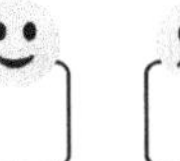  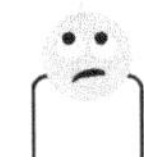 

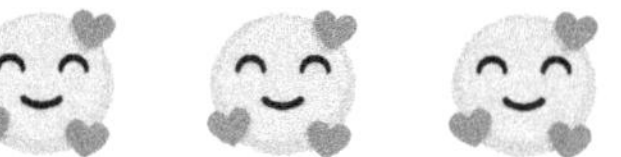

25. Chicken alfredo

  Prep Time : 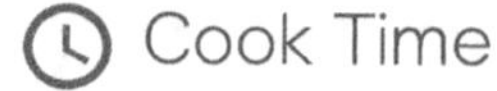 Cook Time : 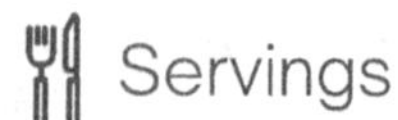 Servings :

Write 5 friends with whom you want to share this dish

Is this dish easy or difficult for you to make?

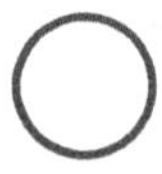 ◯   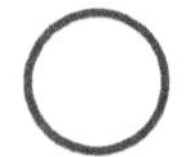 ◯

INGREDIENTS

- 8 oz fettuccine pasta
- 2 boneless, skinless chicken breasts
- 2 tbsp olive oil
- 1 tsp salt
- 1/2 tsp black pepper
- 2 cups heavy cream
- 1 cup grated Parmesan cheese
- 2 cloves garlic, minced
- 2 tbsp unsalted butter
- 2 tbsp chopped fresh parsley (optional)

1. Bring a large pot of salted water to a boil. Cook the fettuccine according to package instructions until al dente. Drain and set aside.

2. Season the chicken breasts with salt and pepper.

3. In a large skillet, heat the olive oil over medium-high heat. Add the chicken and cook for 5-7 minutes per side, until cooked through. Transfer the chicken to a cutting board and let it rest for 5 minutes, then slice or shred it.

4. In the same skillet, reduce the heat to medium and add the heavy cream, Parmesan cheese, and garlic. Whisk constantly until the cheese has melted and the sauce has thickened, about 5 minutes.

5. Reduce the heat to low and stir in the butter until it's melted and the sauce is smooth.

6. Add the cooked fettuccine and shredded chicken to the sauce and toss to coat everything evenly. Serve the chicken alfredo immediately, garnished with chopped fresh parsley if desired.

Tips:
- For extra flavor, add a pinch of nutmeg or lemon zest to the sauce.
- Use grilled or sautéed chicken for a different texture.
- Serve the chicken alfredo with a side salad or garlic bread for a complete meal.

This creamy, cheesy chicken alfredo is sure to be a hit with young teens. The rich, flavorful sauce paired with the tender chicken and pasta makes for a delicious and satisfying dish. Enjoy!

Did you have fun cooking this dish?

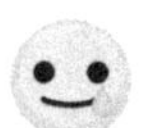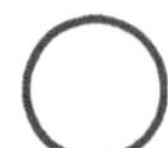 ◯   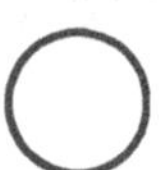 ◯

How would you rate this dish?

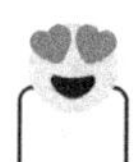 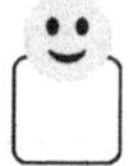   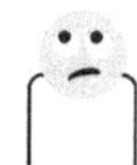 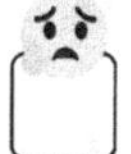

26. BBQ ribs

 *Let's do that and fill in the time here* 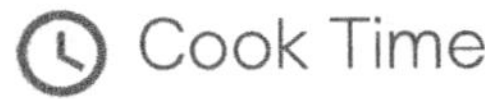 Prep Time : 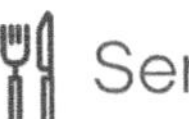 Cook Time : Servings :

Write 5 friends with whom you want to share this dish

....
....
....
....
....

Is this dish easy or difficult for you to make?

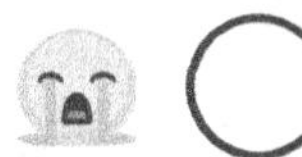 ◯ 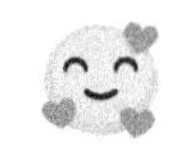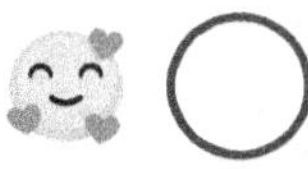 ◯

INGREDIENTS

- 2 lbs baby back ribs or St. Louis-style ribs
- 1 tbsp brown sugar
- 1 tsp smoked paprika
- 1 tsp garlic powder
- 1 tsp onion powder
- 1 tsp salt
- 1/2 tsp black pepper
- 1 cup barbecue sauce (your favorite brand or homemade)

1. Preheat your oven to 300°F.

2. In a small bowl, mix together the brown sugar, smoked paprika, garlic powder, onion powder, salt, and black pepper to make a dry rub.

3. Remove the thin membrane from the back of the ribs by sliding a butter knife under it and peeling it off.

4. Rub the dry rub all over the ribs, making sure to coat both sides.

5. Place the seasoned ribs in a large baking dish or on a rimmed baking sheet. Cover tightly with aluminum foil.

6. Bake the ribs for 2-2.5 hours, until they are tender and the meat is starting to pull away from the bones.

7. Remove the foil and brush the ribs generously with the barbecue sauce.

8. Return the ribs to the oven and bake for an additional 15-20 minutes, until the sauce has caramelized and the ribs are glazed.

9. Let the ribs rest for 5-10 minutes, then cut them into individual portions and serve.

Tips:
- For extra flavor, marinate the ribs in the dry rub for 30 minutes to 1 hour before baking.
- Try different barbecue sauce flavors, like spicy, sweet, or honey mustard.
- Serve the ribs with classic sides like coleslaw, baked beans, or corn on the cob

Did you have fun cooking this dish?

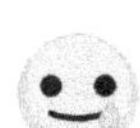 ◯ 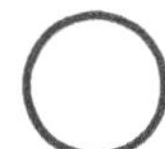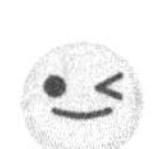 ◯ 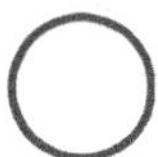

How would you rate this dish?

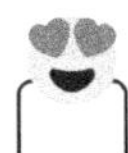 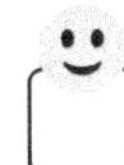 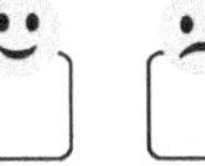 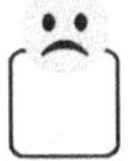 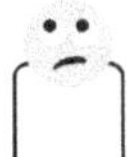 

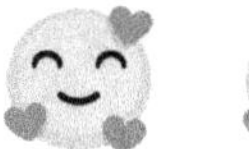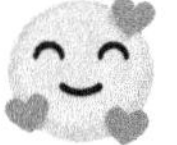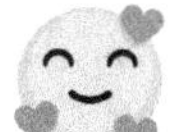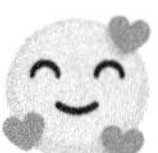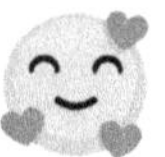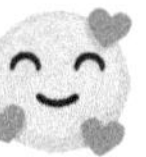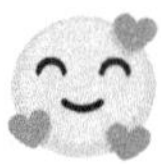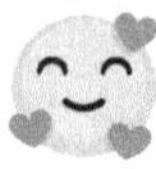

27. Chili cheese dogs

Let's do that and fill in the time here  Prep Time :   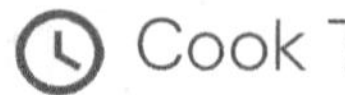 Cook Time :    Servings :

Write 5 friends with whom you want to share this dish

....
....
....
....

INGREDIENTS

- 8 hot dogs
- 8 hot dog buns
- 1 lb ground beef
- 1 onion, diced
- 2 cloves garlic, minced
- 1 packet chili seasoning mix
- 1 (15 oz) can tomato sauce
- 1 (15 oz) can kidney beans, drained and rinsed
- 2 cups shredded cheddar cheese

Did you have fun cooking this dish?

  ◯   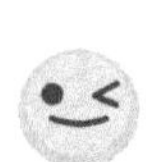 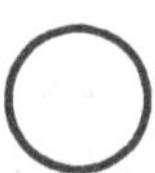 ◯

How would you rate this dish?

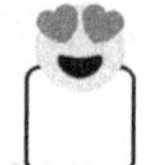 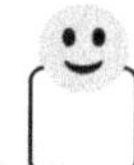 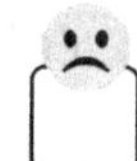 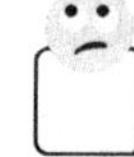 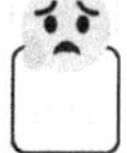

Is this dish easy or difficult for you to make?

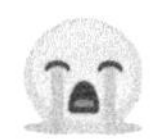 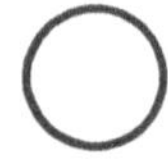 ◯   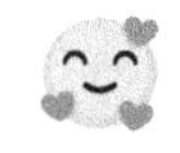 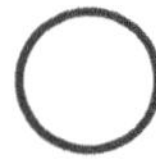 ◯

1. In a large skillet over medium heat, cook the ground beef, onion, and garlic until the beef is browned and the vegetables are softened, about 5-7 minutes. Drain any excess fat.

2. Stir in the chili seasoning mix, tomato sauce, and kidney beans. Simmer the chili for 10-15 minutes, stirring occasionally, until thickened.

3. While the chili is simmering, warm the hot dogs and buns according to package instructions.

4. Place each hot dog in a bun and top with a generous amount of the chili.

5. Sprinkle the shredded cheddar cheese over the chili-topped hot dogs.

6. Serve the chili cheese dogs immediately, while the cheese is melted and gooey.

Tips:
- For extra flavor, add a pinch of cumin, chili powder, or cayenne pepper to the chili.
- Top the chili cheese dogs with diced onions, jalapeños, or a dollop of sour cream.
- Serve the chili cheese dogs with a side of fries or tater tots for a complete meal.

These chili cheese dogs are sure to be a hit with young teens. The combination of the savory hot dog, spicy chili, and melted cheese makes for a delicious and satisfying treat. Enjoy!

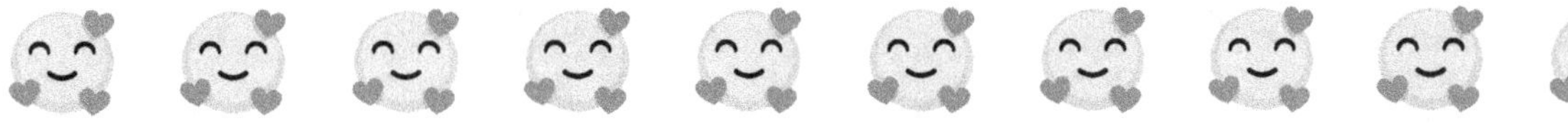

28. Chicken Caesar wrap

 Prep Time : 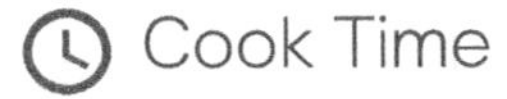

Cook Time : 

Servings :

Write 5 friends with whom you want to share this dish

Is this dish easy or difficult for you to make?

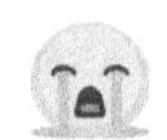 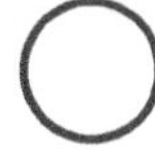 ◯    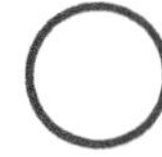 ◯

INGREDIENTS

- 2 boneless, skinless chicken breasts
- 2 tbsp olive oil
- 1 tsp salt
- 1/2 tsp black pepper
- 4 large tortilla wraps
- 2 cups chopped romaine lettuce
- 1 cup shredded Parmesan cheese
- 1/2 cup Caesar salad dressing

1. Preheat your oven to 400°F.

2. Season the chicken breasts with salt and pepper.

3. In a large skillet, heat the olive oil over medium-high heat. Add the chicken and cook for 5-7 minutes per side, until cooked through. Transfer the chicken to a cutting board and let it rest for 5 minutes, then slice or shred it.

4. Lay the tortilla wraps out on a flat surface. Divide the shredded chicken, chopped romaine, Parmesan cheese, and Caesar dressing evenly among the wraps.

5. Fold the bottom of each wrap up over the filling, then fold in the sides and roll up tightly to create a wrap.

6. Wrap the prepared wraps in foil or parchment paper to keep them together.

7. Serve the chicken Caesar wraps immediately, or refrigerate them for up to 4 hours until ready to serve.

Tips:
- For extra crunch, add some croutons or toasted breadcrumbs to the wrap.
- Try using grilled or blackened chicken for a different flavor profile.

These chicken Caesar wraps are sure to be a hit with young teens. They're portable, easy to eat, and packed with delicious flavors that teens love. Serve them as a quick lunch or a satisfying snack. Enjoy!

Did you have fun cooking this dish?

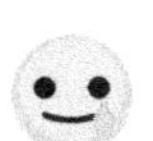 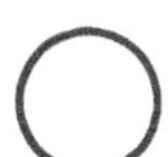 ◯    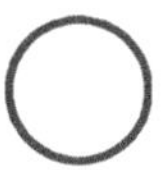 ◯

How would you rate this dish?

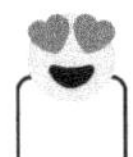 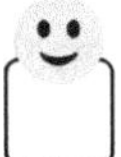 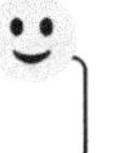  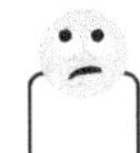 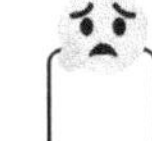 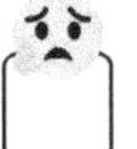

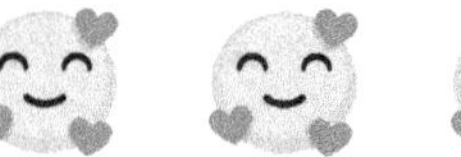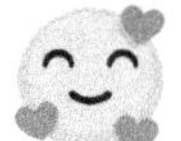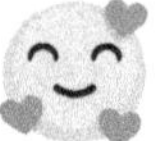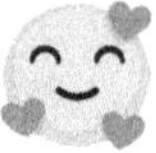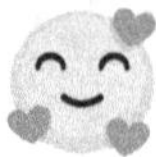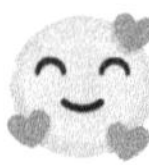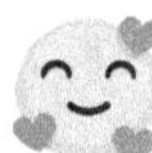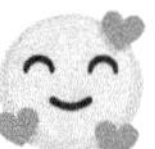

29. Pepperoni rolls

 Prep Time :   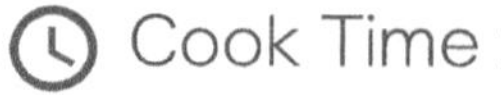 Cook Time :    Servings :

Is this dish easy or difficult for you to make?

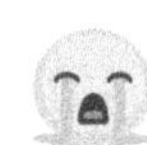 ◯   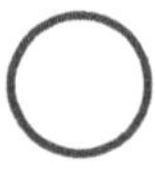 ◯    ◯   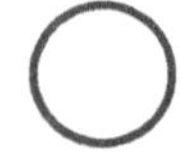 ◯

Write 5 friends with whom you want to share this dish

....
....
....
....
....

INGREDIENTS

- 1 lb pizza dough, store-bought or homemade
- 24 slices of pepperoni
- 8 oz shredded mozzarella cheese
- 1 egg, beaten with 1 tbsp water (for egg wash)

1. Preheat your oven to 400°F. Line a baking sheet with parchment paper.

2. Divide the pizza dough into 12 equal pieces. On a lightly floured surface, roll each piece into a small oval shape, about 4 inches long and 2 inches wide.

3. Place 2 slices of pepperoni and about 2 tablespoons of shredded mozzarella cheese in the center of each dough oval.

4. Fold the dough over the filling to create a half-moon shape, and pinch the edges to seal.

5. Place the filled pepperoni rolls seam-side down on the prepared baking sheet.

6. Brush the tops of the rolls with the egg wash.

7. Bake for 15-18 minutes, until the dough is golden brown and the cheese is melted.

8. Remove the pepperoni rolls from the oven and let them cool for 5 minutes before serving.

Tips:
- For extra flavor, try adding a sprinkle of Italian seasoning or grated Parmesan cheese to the filling.
- Serve the pepperoni rolls warm, with a side of marinara sauce for dipping.
- Experiment with different fillings, such as ham and cheese or spinach and feta.

These homemade pepperoni rolls are sure to be a hit with young teens. They're easy to make, portable, and packed with delicious flavors that teens love. Enjoy!

Did you have fun cooking this dish?

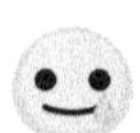 ◯    ◯

How would you rate this dish?

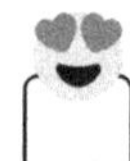   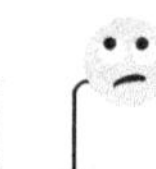 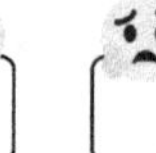

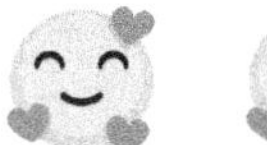 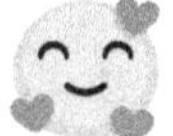 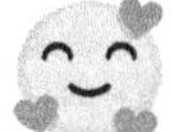 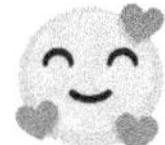 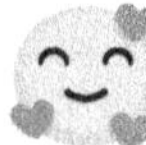 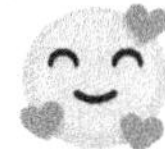 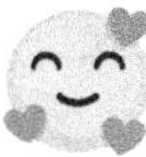 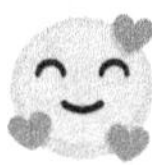 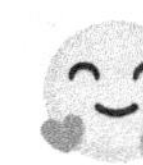 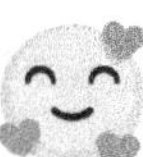

30. Loaded baked potato

Let's do that and fill in the time here

Prep Time :

Cook Time :

Servings :

Write 5 friends with whom you want to share this dish

....

....

....

....

....

INGREDIENTS

- 4 large russet potatoes
- 2 tbsp olive oil
- 1 tsp salt
- 1/2 tsp black pepper
- 1 cup shredded cheddar cheese
- 6 slices bacon, cooked and crumbled
- 4 tbsp sour cream
- 2 tbsp chopped green onions

Is this dish easy or difficult for you to make?

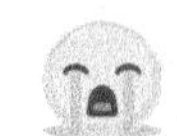 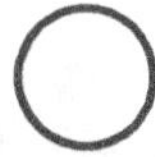 ◯    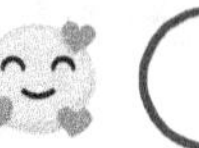 ◯

1. Preheat your oven to 400°F.

2. Scrub the potatoes and prick them several times with a fork. Rub the potatoes with the olive oil and sprinkle with salt and pepper.

3. Place the potatoes directly on the oven rack and bake for 50-60 minutes, until a knife can easily pierce through the center.

4. Remove the potatoes from the oven and let them cool for 5 minutes.

5. Slice each potato in half lengthwise. Use a fork to gently fluff and mash the insides of the potatoes.

6. Top each potato half with shredded cheddar cheese, crumbled bacon, a dollop of sour cream, and a sprinkle of chopped green onions.

7. Serve the loaded baked potatoes immediately, while the cheese is melted and the toppings are warm.

Tips:
- For extra flavor, rub the potatoes with a little butter or olive oil before baking.
- Try different toppings like chili, broccoli, or diced ham.
- Bake the potatoes a day in advance to save time.

These loaded baked potatoes are sure to be a hit with young teens. The combination of the fluffy potato, melted cheese, crispy bacon, and cool sour cream makes for a delicious and satisfying meal or side dish. Enjoy!

Did you have fun cooking this dish?

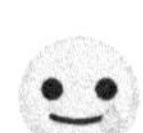 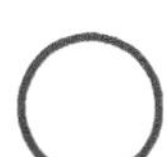 ◯    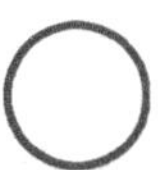 ◯

How would you rate this dish?

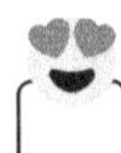 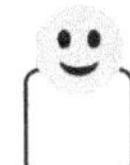 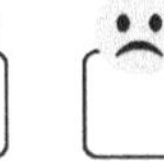 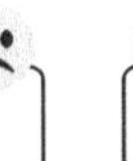 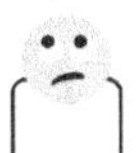 

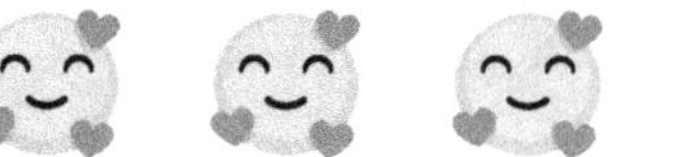

31. Chicken fajitas

Let's do that and fill in the time here  Prep Time :   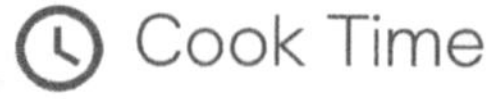 Cook Time :    Servings :

Write 5 friends with whom you want to share this dish

Is this dish easy or difficult for you to make?

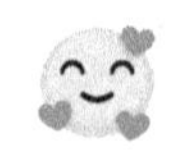 ○   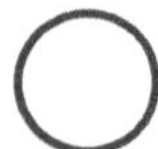 ○

INGREDIENTS

- 1 lb boneless, skinless chicken breasts, sliced into thin strips
- 2 bell peppers (any color), sliced into thin strips
- 1 onion, sliced into thin strips
- 2 tbsp olive oil
- 1 tbsp chili powder
- 1 tsp cumin
- 1 tsp garlic powder
- 1/2 tsp salt
- 1/4 tsp black pepper
- 8-10 flour tortillas
- Toppings (such as shredded cheese, sour cream, guacamole, salsa)

1. In a large skillet or wok, heat the olive oil over medium-high heat.

2. Add the sliced chicken, bell peppers, and onion to the skillet. Sprinkle with the chili powder, cumin, garlic powder, salt, and black pepper.

3. Stir-fry the mixture for 8-10 minutes, or until the chicken is cooked through and the vegetables are tender-crisp.

4. Remove the skillet from the heat and let the fajita mixture cool slightly.

5. Warm the flour tortillas according to package instructions.

6. To assemble the fajitas, place some of the chicken and vegetable mixture into the center of a warm tortilla. Top with your desired toppings, such as shredded cheese, sour cream, guacamole, or salsa.

7. Fold the tortilla over the filling and serve immediately.

Tips:
- For extra flavor, marinate the chicken in a mixture of lime juice, olive oil, and spices for 30 minutes to 1 hour before cooking.
- Offer a variety of toppings so teens can customize their fajitas.

These chicken fajitas are sure to be a hit with young teens. The tender, flavorful chicken and crisp vegetables wrapped in warm tortillas make for a delicious and interactive meal. Enjoy!

Did you have fun cooking this dish?

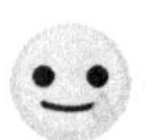 ○    ○

How would you rate this dish?

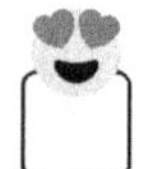 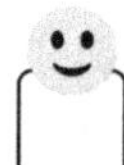  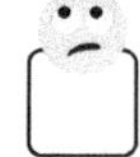 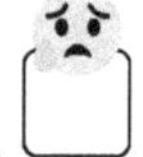

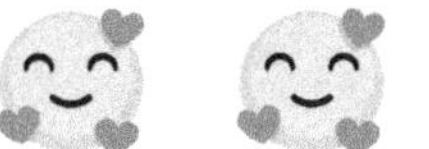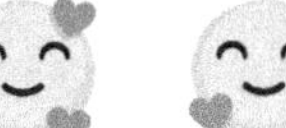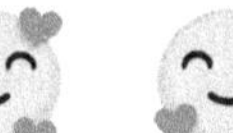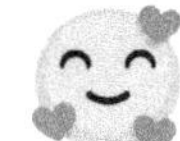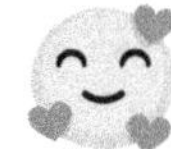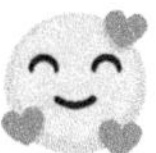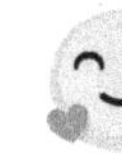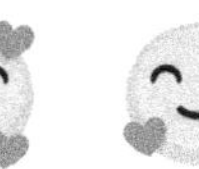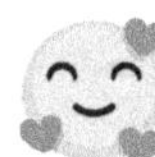

32. Garlic bread

Let's do that and fill in the time here

 Prep Time :　　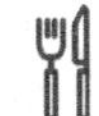 Cook Time :　　Servings :

Write 5 friends with whom you want to share this dish

....
....
....
....
....

INGREDIENTS

- 1 loaf of French or Italian bread, sliced in half lengthwise
- 1/2 cup (1 stick) unsalted butter, softened
- 3 cloves garlic, minced
- 1 tsp dried parsley
- 1/4 tsp salt
- 1/4 tsp black pepper
- 1/4 cup grated Parmesan cheese (optional)

Is this dish easy or difficult for you to make?

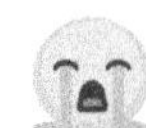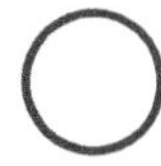 ◯　　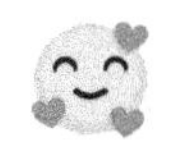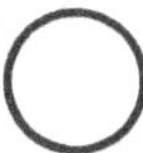 ◯

1. Preheat your oven to 400°F.

2. In a small bowl, mix together the softened butter, minced garlic, dried parsley, salt, and black pepper until well combined.

3. Spread the garlic butter mixture evenly over the cut sides of the bread.

4. If using, sprinkle the grated Parmesan cheese over the buttered bread.

5. Place the bread halves, cut-side up, on a baking sheet.

6. Bake for 10-12 minutes, until the bread is golden brown and the butter is melted.

7. Remove the garlic bread from the oven and let it cool for 2-3 minutes.

8. Cut the bread into slices and serve warm.

Tips:
- For extra flavor, add a pinch of dried oregano or basil to the garlic butter.
- Rub the cut sides of the bread with a halved garlic clove before spreading on the butter.
- Broil the garlic bread for 1-2 minutes at the end to get a crispy, golden top.

This homemade garlic bread is sure to be a hit with young teens. The garlicky, buttery flavor paired with the crispy, toasted bread makes for a delicious and irresistible side dish. Enjoy!

Did you have fun cooking this dish?

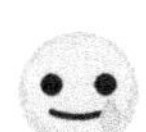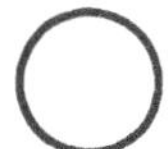 ◯　　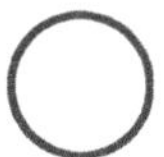 ◯

How would you rate this dish?

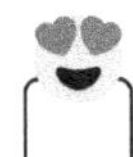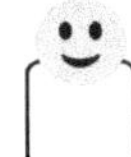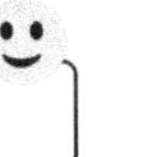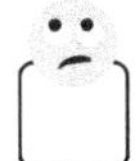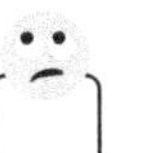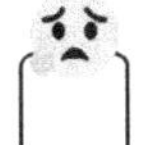

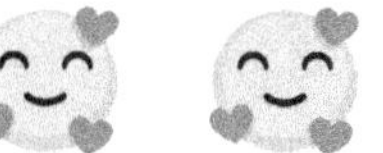 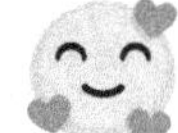 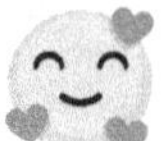 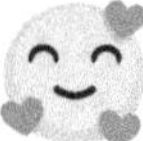 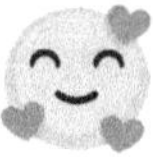 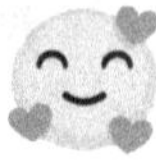 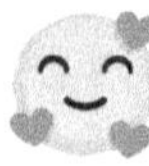 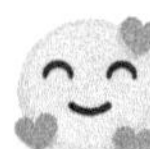 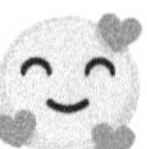

33. Cheese pizza rolls

 Prep Time : 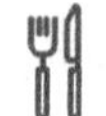 Cook Time : Servings :

Is this dish easy or difficult for you to make?

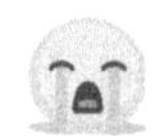 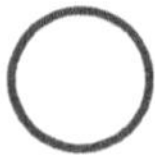 ◯    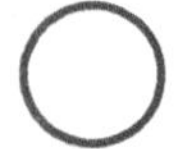 ◯

Write 5 friends with whom you want to share this dish

....

....

....

....

....

INGREDIENTS

- 1 (8 oz) can refrigerated crescent roll dough
- 1/2 cup shredded mozzarella cheese
- 1/4 cup grated Parmesan cheese
- 1/4 cup mini pepperoni slices (optional)
- 1/4 cup pizza sauce, plus more for dipping
- 1 teaspoon dried oregano

1. Preheat your oven to 375°F. Line a baking sheet with parchment paper.

2. Unroll the crescent roll dough and separate it into 8 triangles.

3. In a small bowl, mix together the mozzarella cheese, Parmesan cheese, and pepperoni (if using).

4. Place a heaping tablespoon of the cheese mixture onto the wide end of each crescent roll triangle.

5. Fold the pointed end of the triangle over the filling and roll it up towards the wide end, enclosing the filling completely.

6. Place the rolled-up pizza rolls seam-side down on the prepared baking sheet.

7. In a small bowl, mix together the 1/4 cup of pizza sauce and the dried oregano.

8. Brush the tops of the pizza rolls with the seasoned pizza sauce.

9. Bake for 12-15 minutes, until the rolls are golden brown.

10. Serve the warm pizza rolls with additional pizza sauce for dipping.

Tips:
- Use mini pepperoni for a kid-friendly size, or leave them out for a simpler cheese filling.
- Experiment with different cheese combinations, such as cheddar or provolone.

Did you have fun cooking this dish?

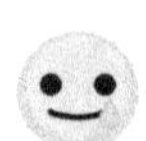 ◯    ◯

How would you rate this dish?

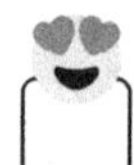 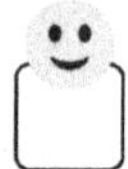  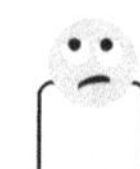 

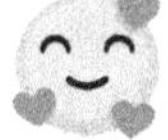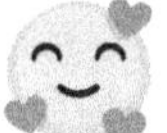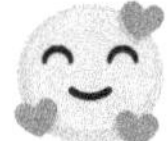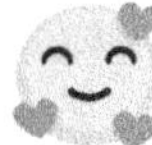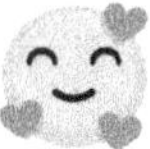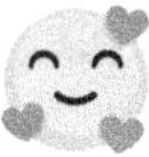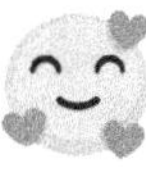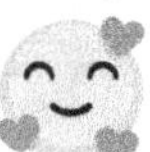

34. Chicken sandwich

Let's do that and fill in the time here

 Prep Time :　　　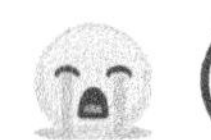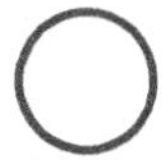 Cook Time :　　　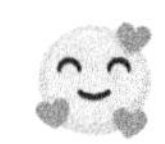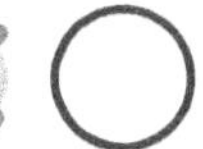 Servings :

Is this dish easy or difficult for you to make?

○　　　○

Write 5 friends with whom you want to share this dish

....

....

....

....

....

INGREDIENTS

- 2 boneless, skinless chicken breasts
- 1 cup all-purpose flour
- 1 tsp salt
- 1/2 tsp black pepper
- 2 eggs, beaten
- 1 cup panko breadcrumbs
- Vegetable oil for frying
- 4 hamburger buns, split
- Lettuce, tomato, and pickle slices (optional toppings)

For the Sauce:
- 1/2 cup mayonnaise
- 2 tbsp Dijon mustard
- 1 tbsp honey
- 1 tsp apple cider vinegar
- 1/4 tsp garlic powder
- 1/4 tsp paprika

1. Pound the chicken breasts between two sheets of plastic wrap or parchment paper to an even 1/2-inch thickness.

2. Set up a breading station with three shallow dishes: one with the flour, salt, and pepper mixed together; one with the beaten eggs; and one with the panko breadcrumbs.

3. Dredge the chicken breasts in the flour mixture, dip them in the egg, and then coat them in the panko breadcrumbs, pressing gently to adhere.

4. In a large skillet or Dutch oven, heat 1-2 inches of vegetable oil to 350°F.

5. Carefully add the breaded chicken to the hot oil and fry for 3-4 minutes per side, until golden brown and cooked through.

6. Transfer the fried chicken to a paper towel-lined plate to drain any excess oil.

7. In a small bowl, mix together all the sauce ingredients.

8. Spread the sauce on the top and bottom buns. Place the fried chicken on the bottom buns and top with lettuce, tomato, and pickle slices, if desired. Serve the crispy chicken sandwiches immediately.

Tips:
- For extra crunch, let the breaded chicken sit in the refrigerator for 30 minutes before frying.
- Bake the chicken at 400°F for 20-25 minutes instead of frying for a healthier option.

Did you have fun cooking this dish?

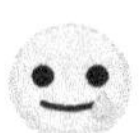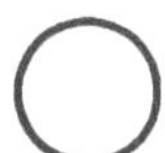 ○　　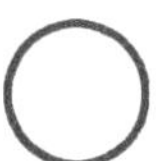 ○

How would you rate this dish?

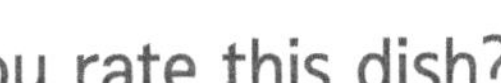

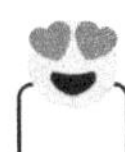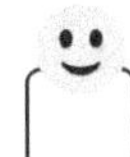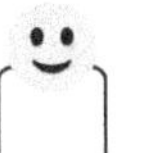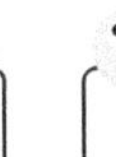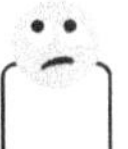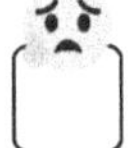

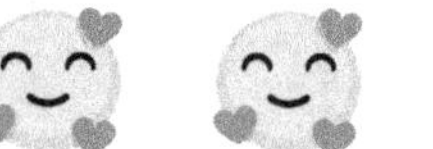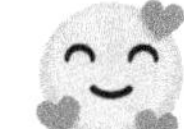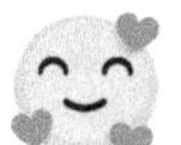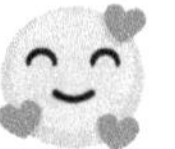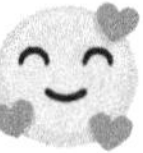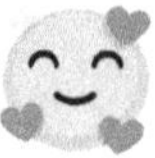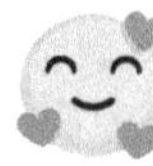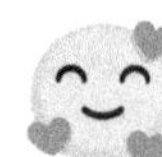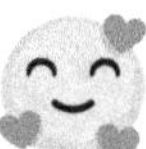

35. Beef burrito

  Prep Time : 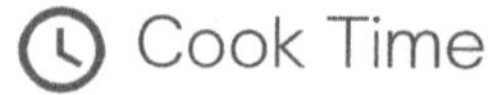 Cook Time : 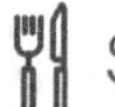 Servings :

Write 5 friends with whom you want to share this dish

....
....
....
....
....

INGREDIENTS

- 1 lb ground beef
- 1 packet taco seasoning
- 1/2 cup water
- 8 large flour tortillas
- 1 cup cooked rice
- 1 (15 oz) can black beans, drained and rinsed
- 1 cup shredded cheddar or Mexican blend cheese
- Salsa, sour cream, and other desired toppings

Is this dish easy or difficult for you to make?

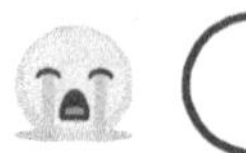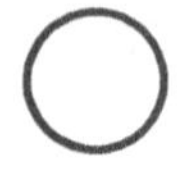 ◯   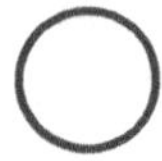 ◯

1. In a large skillet, cook the ground beef over medium heat until browned and crumbled, 5-7 minutes. Drain any excess fat.

2. Stir in the taco seasoning and water. Simmer for 5 minutes, stirring occasionally, until the sauce has thickened.

3. Warm the tortillas according to package instructions to make them pliable.

4. Lay a tortilla flat and layer with 2-3 tablespoons of the seasoned ground beef, 2-3 tablespoons of rice, 2-3 tablespoons of black beans, and 2-3 tablespoons of shredded cheese.

5. Fold the bottom of the tortilla up over the filling, then fold in the sides and continue rolling up tightly into a burrito shape.

6. Place the burrito seam-side down on a plate. Repeat with the remaining tortillas and fillings.

7. Serve the beef burritos warm, with salsa, sour cream, and any other desired toppings on the side.

Tips:
- Use mild taco seasoning for a less spicy flavor.
- Customize the fillings to your teen's preferences, such as adding diced tomatoes, lettuce, or guacamole.
- Wrap individual burritos in foil to keep them warm and portable.

Enjoy these easy and delicious beef burritos!

Did you have fun cooking this dish?

 ◯   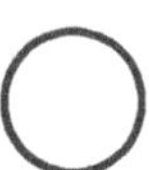 ◯

How would you rate this dish?

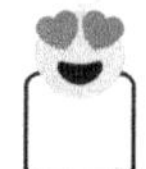 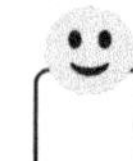  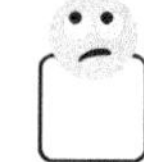 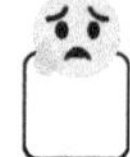

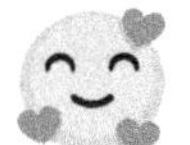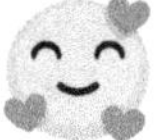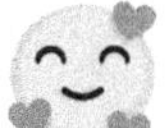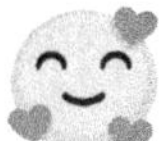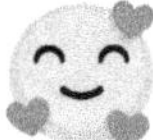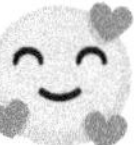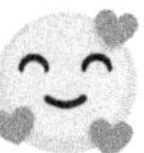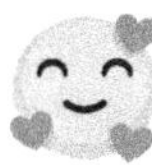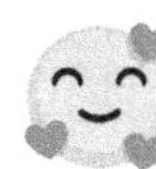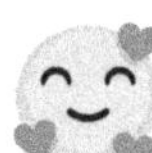

36. Corn dogs

Let's do that and fill in the time here 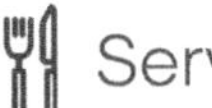 Prep Time :   Cook Time :   Servings :

Write 5 friends with whom you want to share this dish
....
....
....
....
....

Is this dish easy or difficult for you to make?

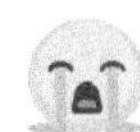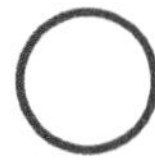 ◯   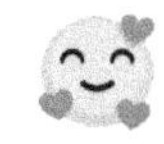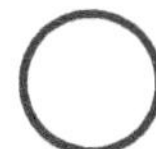 ◯

INGREDIENTS

- 1 cup all-purpose flour
- 1/2 cup yellow cornmeal
- 2 tablespoons white sugar
- 1 teaspoon baking powder
- 1/2 teaspoon salt
- 1 egg
- 3/4 cup milk
- 8 hot dogs or mini corn dog sausages
- Vegetable oil for frying

1. In a medium bowl, whisk together the flour, cornmeal, sugar, baking powder, and salt.

2. In a separate bowl, beat the egg and then stir in the milk.

3. Pour the milk mixture into the dry ingredients and stir just until combined (do not overmix).

4. Insert wooden skewers or popsicle sticks into the hot dogs.

5. Heat 2-3 inches of vegetable oil in a large pot or Dutch oven to 350°F.

6. Dip the hot dogs into the corn dog batter, coating them completely.

7. Carefully lower the battered hot dogs into the hot oil and fry for 2-3 minutes, turning occasionally, until golden brown.

8. Remove the corn dogs from the oil and place on a paper towel-lined plate to drain excess oil.

9. Serve the corn dogs warm, with ketchup, mustard, or other dipping sauces on the side.

Tips:
- Use mini corn dog sausages for a kid-friendly size.
- Let the batter rest for 10-15 minutes before dipping the hot dogs to help it thicken up.
- Adjust the sugar to taste if desired - you can reduce it for a less sweet batter.

Did you have fun cooking this dish?

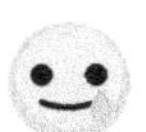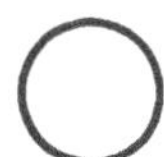 ◯   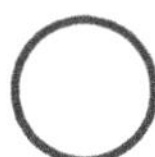 ◯

How would you rate this dish?

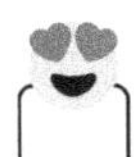 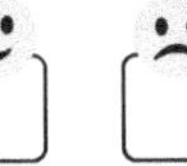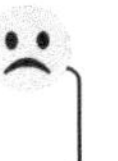 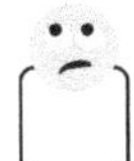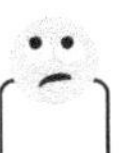 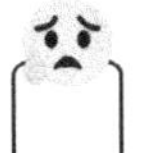

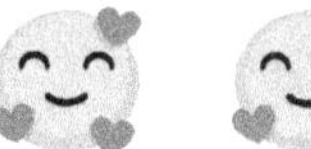 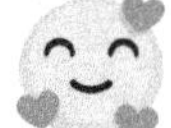 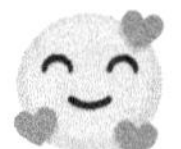 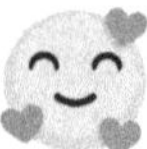 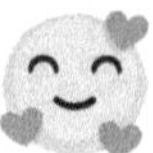 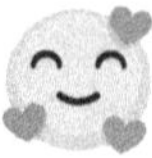 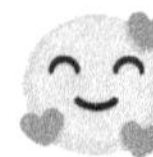  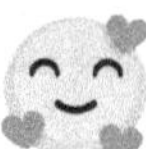

37. Fried pickles

Let's do that and fill in the time here  Prep Time :   Cook Time :   Servings :

Write 5 friends with whom you want to share this dish
....
....
....
....
....

Is this dish easy or difficult for you to make?

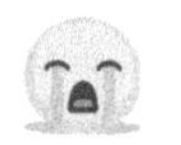 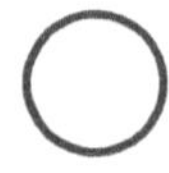 ◯   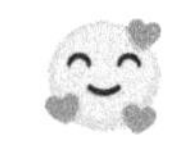 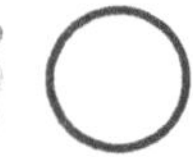 ◯

INGREDIENTS

- 1 cup all-purpose flour
- 1 teaspoon garlic powder
- 1 teaspoon paprika
- 1/2 teaspoon cayenne pepper
- 1/2 teaspoon salt
- 1 cup buttermilk
- 1 (16 oz) jar dill pickle chips, drained and patted dry
- Vegetable oil for frying
- Ranch dressing or other dipping sauce for serving

1. In a shallow bowl, whisk together the flour, garlic powder, paprika, cayenne, and salt.

2. Pour the buttermilk into a separate shallow bowl.

3. Dip the pickle chips into the buttermilk, allowing any excess to drip off. Then dredge the pickles in the seasoned flour, coating them completely.

4. In a large skillet or Dutch oven, heat 1-2 inches of vegetable oil to 350°F.

5. Working in batches, carefully add the breaded pickle chips to the hot oil and fry for 2-3 minutes until golden brown and crispy.

6. Transfer the fried pickles to a paper towel-lined plate to drain any excess oil.

7. Serve the fried pickles immediately, with ranch dressing or your favorite dipping sauce on the side.

Did you have fun cooking this dish?

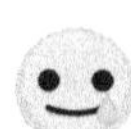 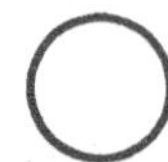 ◯   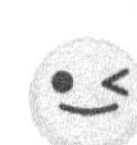 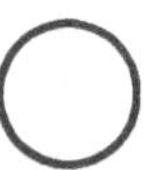 ◯

How would you rate this dish?

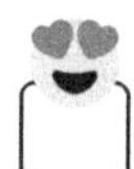   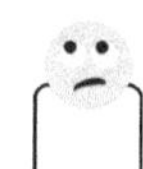 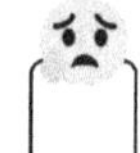

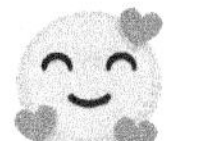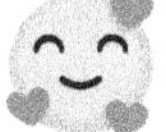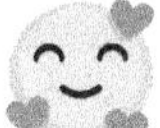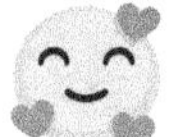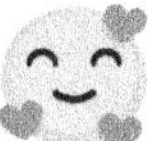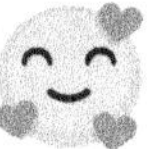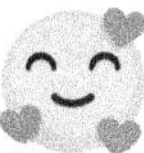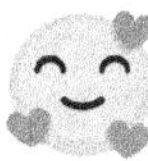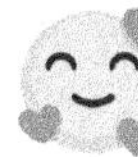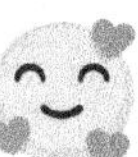

38. Cheese sticks

Let's do that and fill in the time here

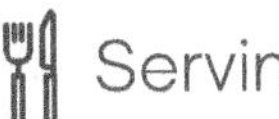 Prep Time :

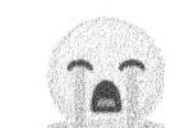 Cook Time :

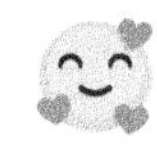 Servings :

Is this dish easy or difficult for you to make?

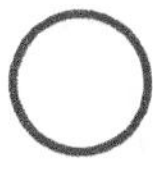 ◯   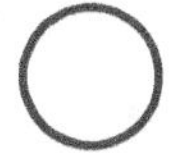 ◯

Write 5 friends with whom you want to share this dish

....
....
....
....
....

INGREDIENTS

- 1 (8 oz) block of mozzarella cheese, cut into 1/2-inch thick sticks
- 1 cup all-purpose flour
- 2 eggs, beaten
- 1 cup panko breadcrumbs
- 1/2 cup grated Parmesan cheese
- 1 teaspoon dried oregano
- 1/2 teaspoon garlic powder
- 1/4 teaspoon salt
- Marinara sauce or ranch dressing for dipping

Did you have fun cooking this dish?

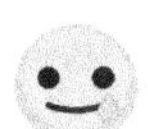  ◯   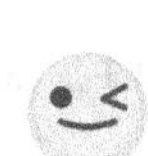 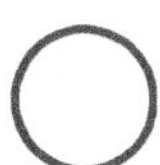 ◯

How would you rate this dish?

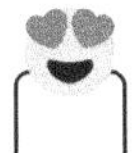 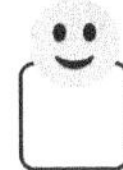 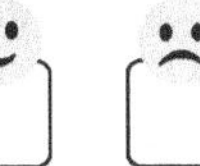 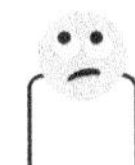 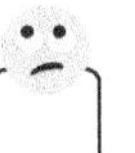 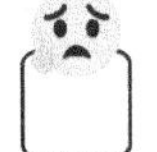

1. Preheat your oven to 400°F. Line a baking sheet with parchment paper.

2. Set up a breading station with three shallow dishes:
   - In the first dish, place the all-purpose flour.
   - In the second dish, place the beaten eggs.
   - In the third dish, mix together the panko breadcrumbs, Parmesan cheese, oregano, garlic powder, and salt.

3. Dip each cheese stick first in the flour, coating all sides, then in the beaten egg, and finally in the breadcrumb mixture, pressing gently to help the crumbs adhere.

4. Place the breaded cheese sticks on the prepared baking sheet, making sure they are not touching.

5. Bake for 8-10 minutes, or until the cheese sticks are golden brown and crispy.

6. Serve the warm cheese sticks immediately with marinara sauce or ranch dressing for dipping.

Tips:
- Use low-moisture mozzarella cheese for best results.
- Chill the breaded cheese sticks for 30 minutes before baking to help them hold their shape.
- For extra crispiness, spray the cheese sticks lightly with cooking spray before baking.
- Adjust the baking time as needed, depending on the thickness of your cheese sticks.

39. Chicken noodle soup

  Prep Time :   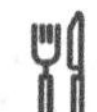 Cook Time :   Servings :

Is this dish easy or difficult for you to make?

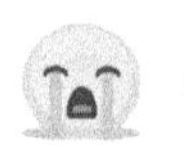 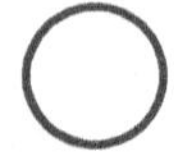 ◯   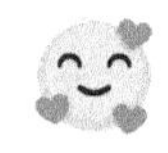 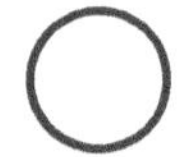 ◯

Write 5 friends with whom you want to share this dish

....

....

....

....

INGREDIENTS

- 1 lb boneless, skinless chicken breasts
- 8 cups chicken broth
- 2 carrots, peeled and sliced
- 2 celery stalks, sliced
- 1 onion, diced
- 2 cloves garlic, minced
- 2 cups egg noodles
- 2 tablespoons chopped fresh parsley
- Salt and pepper to taste

1. In a large pot or Dutch oven, place the chicken breasts and pour in the chicken broth. Bring the broth to a boil over high heat.

2. Reduce the heat to medium-low, cover the pot, and let the chicken simmer for 15-20 minutes, or until the chicken is cooked through.

3. Remove the chicken from the pot and set it aside to cool slightly. Once cool enough to handle, shred or chop the chicken into bite-sized pieces.

4. Return the shredded chicken to the pot with the broth.

5. Add the sliced carrots, celery, diced onion, and minced garlic to the pot. Bring the soup back to a simmer and cook for 10-15 minutes, or until the vegetables are tender.

6. Stir in the egg noodles and cook for an additional 5-7 minutes, or until the noodles are tender.

7. Remove the pot from the heat and stir in the chopped fresh parsley. Season with salt and pepper to taste.

8. Serve the chicken noodle soup hot, with crackers or bread on the side.

Tips:
- Use low-sodium chicken broth to control the sodium content.
- Customize the vegetables to your teen's preferences, such as adding peas or corn.
- For a heartier meal, serve the soup with a side salad or grilled cheese sandwich.

Did you have fun cooking this dish?

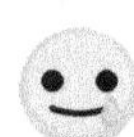  ◯   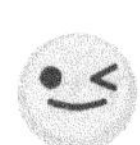 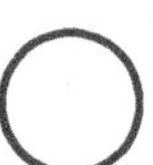 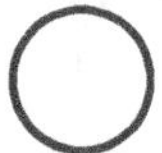 ◯

How would you rate this dish?

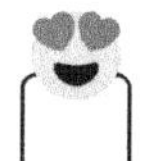 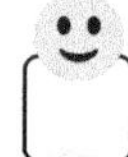  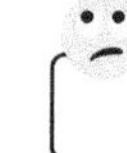 

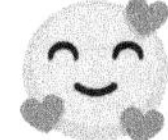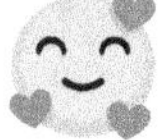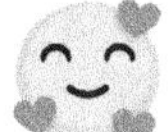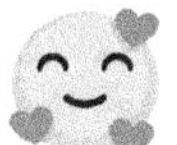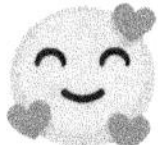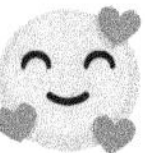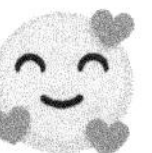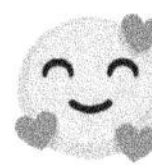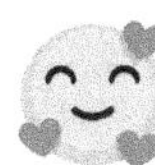

40. Philly cheesesteak

Let's do that and fill in the time here  Prep Time :   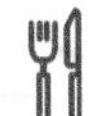 Cook Time :   Servings :

Write 5 friends with whom you want to share this dish
....
....
....
....
....

Is this dish easy or difficult for you to make?

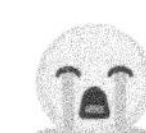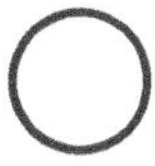 ◯   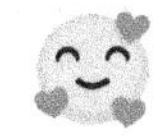 ◯

INGREDIENTS

- 1 lb thinly sliced beef sirloin or ribeye
- 2 tablespoons olive oil
- 1 large onion, thinly sliced
- 1 green bell pepper, thinly sliced
- 8 oz sliced mushrooms (optional)
- 4 hoagie or sub rolls, split lengthwise
- 8 slices provolone cheese

1. Heat the olive oil in a large skillet or griddle over medium-high heat.

2. Add the sliced beef and cook, stirring frequently, until the beef is browned and cooked through, about 5-7 minutes. Transfer the beef to a plate and set aside.

3. In the same skillet, add the sliced onions, bell pepper, and mushrooms (if using). Cook, stirring occasionally, until the vegetables are tender and lightly caramelized, about 8-10 minutes.

4. Return the cooked beef to the skillet with the vegetables. Stir to combine and heat through.

5. Preheat your oven's broiler.

6. Place the split hoagie rolls on a baking sheet. Top each roll with the beef and vegetable mixture, then top with 2 slices of provolone cheese.

7. Broil the Philly cheesesteaks for 2-3 minutes, or until the cheese is melted and bubbly.

8. Serve the Philly cheesesteaks immediately, while hot.

Tips:
- Use thinly sliced beef to ensure it cooks quickly and stays tender.
- Customize the toppings to your teen's preferences, such as adding mushrooms or using American cheese instead of provolone.
- Serve with a side of fries or a fresh salad for a complete meal.

Did you have fun cooking this dish?

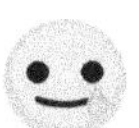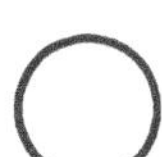 ◯   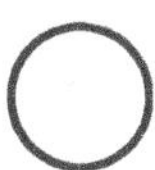 ◯

How would you rate this dish?

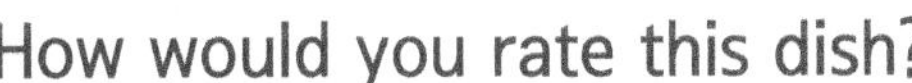
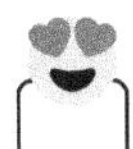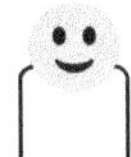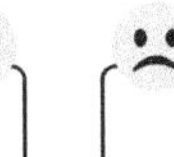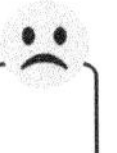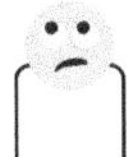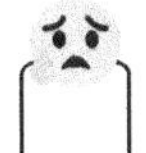

41. Ham and cheese panini

 Prep Time :

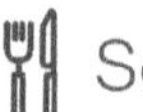 Cook Time :

Servings :

Write 5 friends with whom you want to share this dish

....

....

....

....

....

INGREDIENTS

- 8 slices of bread (such as sourdough or ciabatta)
- 8 slices of ham
- 8 slices of Swiss or cheddar cheese
- 2 tablespoons butter, softened

Is this dish easy or difficult for you to make?

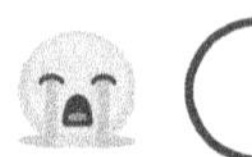 ◯   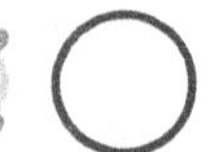 ◯

1. Preheat your panini press or grill pan over medium heat.

2. Lay the 8 slices of bread out on a clean work surface. Place 1-2 slices of ham and 1-2 slices of cheese on 4 of the bread slices.

3. Top the ham and cheese with the remaining 4 bread slices to create 4 sandwiches.

4. Spread the softened butter evenly on the outside of each sandwich.

5. Place the sandwiches in the preheated panini press or grill pan. Close the lid and cook for 3-5 minutes, or until the bread is golden brown and the cheese is melted.

6. Carefully remove the panini from the press using a spatula. Let them cool for 1-2 minutes before serving.

Tips:
- Use a variety of cheeses, such as cheddar, Swiss, provolone, or Gruyère, for different flavor combinations.
- Add other fillings like tomato, spinach, or pesto for extra flavor.
- Press down on the panini with a heavy object, like a cast-iron skillet, to get those signature grill marks.
- Serve the panini with a side of chips, a salad, or a cup of tomato soup for a complete meal.

Did you have fun cooking this dish?

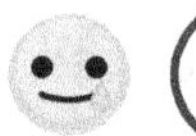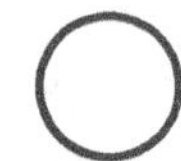 ◯   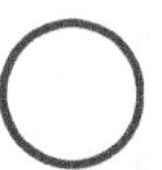 ◯

How would you rate this dish?

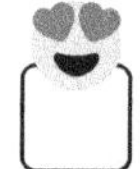 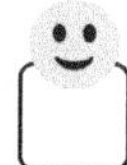  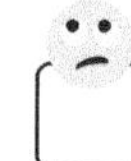 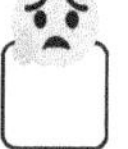

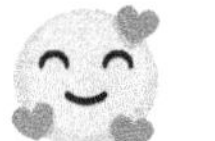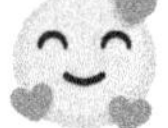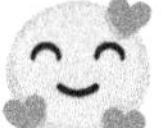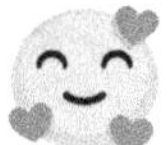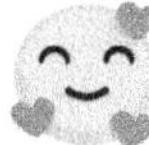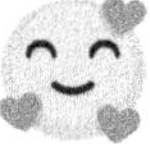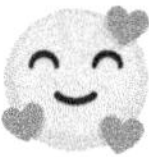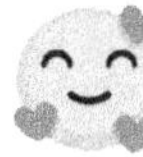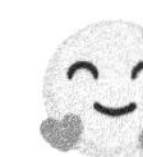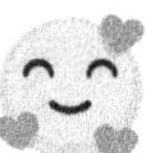

42. BBQ chicken pizza

Let's do that and fill in the time here

 Prep Time : Cook Time : Servings :

Write 5 friends with whom you want to share this dish ....

Is this dish easy or difficult for you to make?

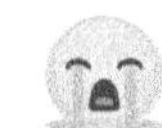 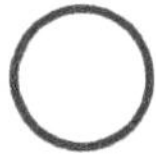 ◯   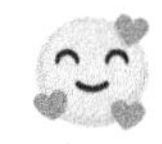 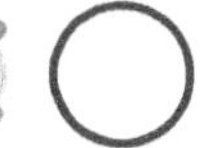 ◯

INGREDIENTS

- 1 lb boneless, skinless chicken breasts, cubed
- 1 tablespoon olive oil
- 1 cup barbecue sauce, divided
- 1 (13.8 oz) package refrigerated pizza dough
- 1 cup shredded mozzarella cheese
- 1/2 cup shredded cheddar cheese
- 1/4 cup thinly sliced red onion
- 2 tablespoons chopped fresh cilantro (optional)

1. Preheat your oven to 400°F. Grease a large baking sheet or pizza pan.

2. In a skillet, heat the olive oil over medium-high heat. Add the cubed chicken and cook until browned and cooked through, about 6-8 minutes.

3. Reduce the heat to low and stir in 1/2 cup of the barbecue sauce. Simmer for 2-3 minutes, then remove from heat.

4. Roll or stretch the pizza dough out to fit the prepared baking sheet or pizza pan.

5. Spread the remaining 1/2 cup of barbecue sauce evenly over the dough.

6. Top the pizza with the cooked BBQ chicken, mozzarella cheese, cheddar cheese, and sliced red onion.

7. Bake for 12-15 minutes, or until the crust is golden brown and the cheese is melted and bubbly.

8. Remove the pizza from the oven and sprinkle with the chopped fresh cilantro, if using.

9. Slice and serve the BBQ chicken pizza warm.

Tips:
- Use a pre-made pizza crust or naan bread for an even quicker assembly.
- Customize the toppings to your teen's preferences, such as adding pineapple or bacon.
- Serve with a side salad or veggie sticks for a balanced meal.

Did you have fun cooking this dish?

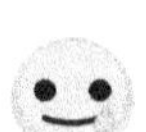 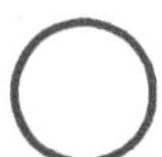 ◯    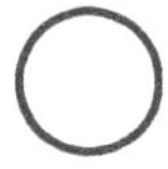 ◯

How would you rate this dish?

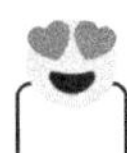 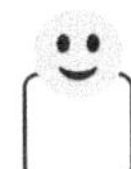 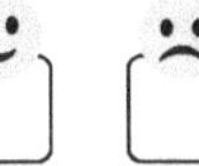  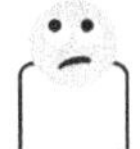 

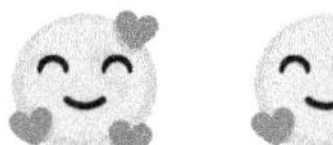 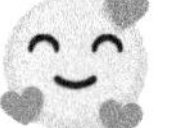 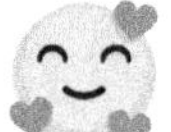 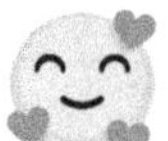 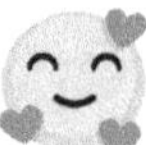 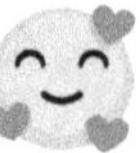 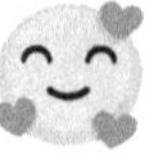 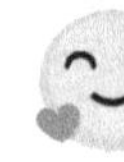  

43. Bacon cheeseburger

Let's do that and fill in the time here  Prep Time :   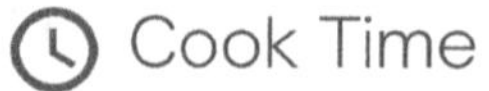 Cook Time :   Servings :

Write 5 friends with whom you want to share this dish ....

Is this dish easy or difficult for you to make?

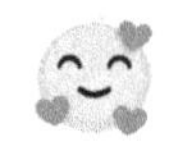 ◯   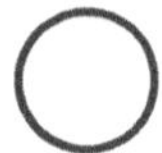 ◯

INGREDIENTS

- 1 lb ground beef
- 1 teaspoon salt
- 1/2 teaspoon black pepper
- 4 slices cheddar or American cheese
- 4 hamburger buns, split
- 8 slices cooked bacon
- Lettuce, tomato, onion, and other desired toppings

1. Preheat your grill or grill pan to medium-high heat.

2. In a bowl, gently mix the ground beef with the salt and pepper until just combined. Divide the mixture into 4 equal portions and shape them into patties, being careful not to overwork the meat.

3. Grill the burger patties for 3-4 minutes per side, or until they reach your desired level of doneness.

4. During the last minute of cooking, place a slice of cheese on top of each patty to melt.

5. Toast the hamburger buns on the grill for 1-2 minutes, until lightly golden.

6. Place the cheeseburger patties on the bottom buns, then top each with 2 slices of cooked bacon.

7. Add any desired toppings, such as lettuce, tomato, onion, pickles, or condiments.

8. Place the top buns on the burgers and serve immediately.

Tips:
- Use lean ground beef to keep the burgers from being too greasy.
- Cook the bacon in advance to make assembly quicker.
- Offer a variety of toppings and condiments so teens can customize their burgers.
- Serve the bacon cheeseburgers with a side of fries or a fresh salad for a complete meal.

Did you have fun cooking this dish?

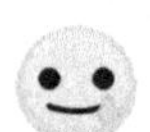 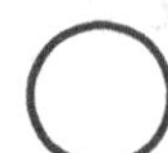 ◯    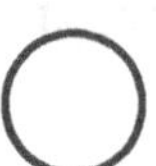 ◯

How would you rate this dish?

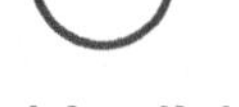

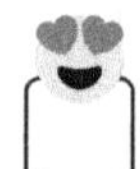 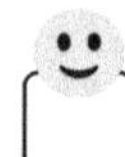 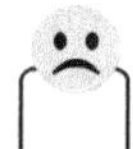 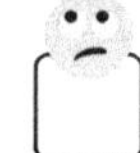 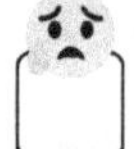

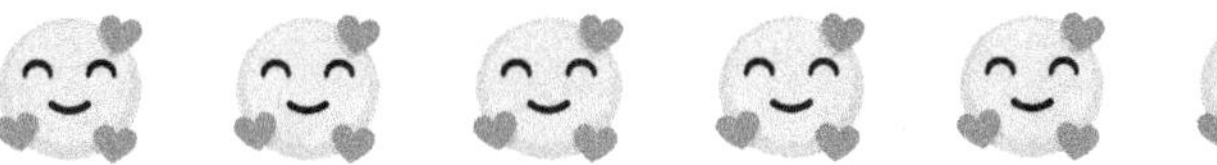

44. Chicken pot pie

 Prep Time :    Cook Time :   Servings :

Is this dish easy or difficult for you to make?

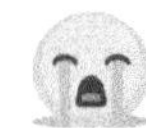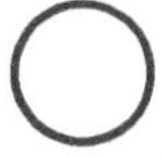 ◯   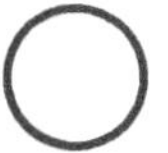 ◯

Write 5 friends with whom you want to share this dish

....

....

....

....

....

INGREDIENTS

- 1 lb boneless, skinless chicken breasts, cubed
- 2 tablespoons olive oil
- 1 onion, diced
- 2 carrots, peeled and diced
- 2 celery stalks, diced
- 2 cloves garlic, minced
- 1/4 cup all-purpose flour
- 2 cups chicken broth
- 1 cup milk
- 1 teaspoon dried thyme
- 1/2 teaspoon dried sage
- Salt and pepper to taste
- 1 (15 oz) package refrigerated pie crusts

Did you have fun cooking this dish?

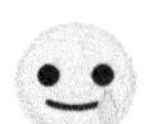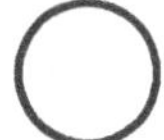 ◯   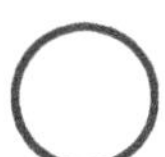 ◯

How would you rate this dish?

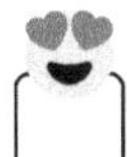 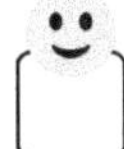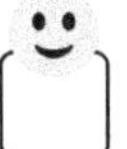  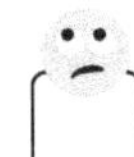 

1. Preheat your oven to 400°F.

2. In a large skillet, heat the olive oil over medium-high heat. Add the cubed chicken and cook until browned, about 5-7 minutes. Remove the chicken from the skillet and set aside.

3. In the same skillet, sauté the onion, carrots, celery, and garlic until softened, about 5 minutes.

4. Sprinkle the flour over the vegetable mixture and stir to coat. Cook for 1 minute.

5. Gradually whisk in the chicken broth and milk. Bring the mixture to a simmer and cook until thickened, about 5 minutes.

6. Stir in the cooked chicken, thyme, sage, salt, and pepper. Taste and adjust seasonings as needed.

7. Unroll one of the pie crusts and place it in a 9-inch pie dish, pressing it into the sides and bottom.

8. Pour the chicken and vegetable mixture into the pie dish.

9. Unroll the second pie crust and place it over the filling. Crimp the edges to seal and cut a few slits in the top crust to allow steam to escape.

10. Bake for 30-35 minutes, or until the crust is golden brown and the filling is bubbly.

11. Let the pot pie cool for 10-15 minutes before slicing and serving

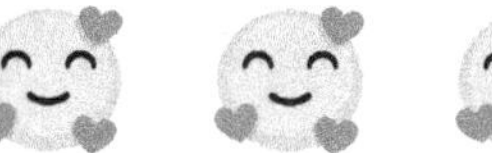 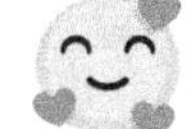 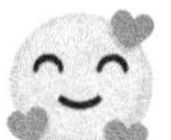 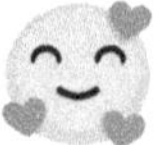 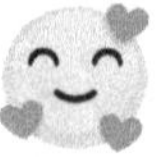 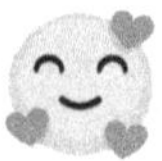 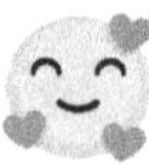  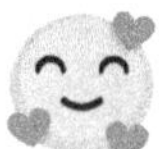

45. Chicken fried rice

 Prep Time : 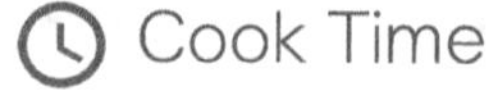 Cook Time : 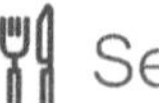 Servings :

Write 5 friends with whom you want to share this dish

....

....

....

....

Is this dish easy or difficult for you to make?

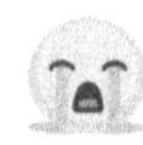 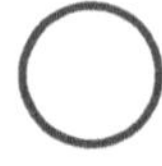 ◯   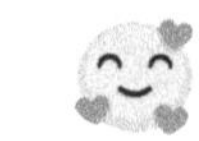 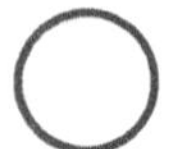 ◯

INGREDIENTS

- 2 cups cooked white rice, chilled
- 2 tablespoons vegetable oil
- 1 lb boneless, skinless chicken breasts, cut into 1-inch pieces
- 1 cup frozen peas and carrots, thawed
- 2 eggs, lightly beaten
- 2 tablespoons soy sauce
- 1 teaspoon sesame oil
- 2 green onions, thinly sliced
- Salt and pepper to taste

1. Heat the vegetable oil in a large skillet or wok over medium-high heat.

2. Add the chicken pieces and cook, stirring occasionally, until the chicken is cooked through, about 5-7 minutes. Transfer the chicken to a plate and set aside.

3. In the same skillet, add the thawed peas and carrots. Cook for 2-3 minutes, stirring frequently, until heated through.

4. Push the vegetables to the side of the skillet and pour the beaten eggs into the empty space. Scramble the eggs, stirring frequently, until cooked through, about 2-3 minutes.

5. Add the cooked chicken back to the skillet, along with the chilled rice, soy sauce, and sesame oil. Stir everything together until well combined and heated through, about 3-5 minutes.

6. Remove the skillet from the heat and stir in the sliced green onions.

7. Season the chicken fried rice with salt and pepper to taste.

8. Serve the fried rice hot, garnished with additional green onions if desired.

Enjoy this tasty and easy-to-make chicken fried rice!

Did you have fun cooking this dish?

 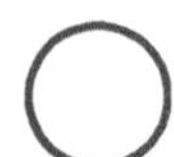 ◯   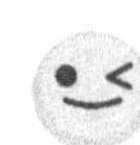 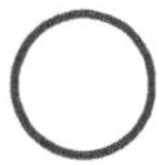 ◯

How would you rate this dish?

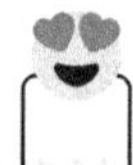 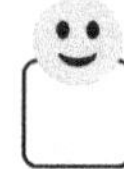 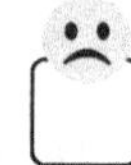 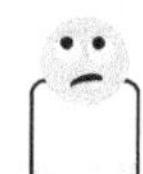 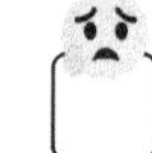 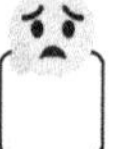

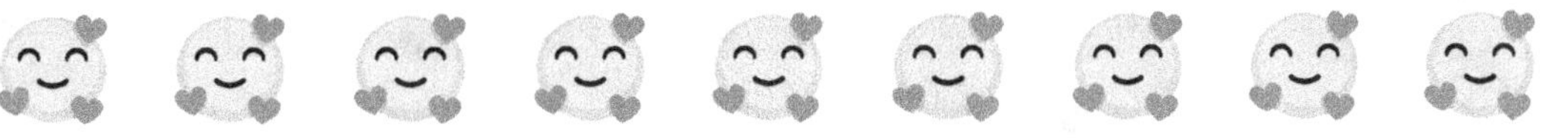

46. Beef nachos

 Prep Time :   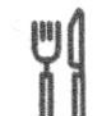 Cook Time :   Servings :

Write 5 friends with whom you want to share this dish

....
....
....
....

Is this dish easy or difficult for you to make?

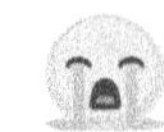 ○   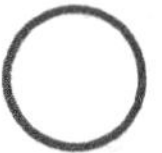 ○

INGREDIENTS

- 1 lb ground beef
- 1 packet taco seasoning
- 1/2 cup water
- 1 (13 oz) bag tortilla chips
- 2 cups shredded cheddar cheese
- 1 (15 oz) can black beans, drained and rinsed
- 1 cup diced tomatoes
- 1/2 cup sliced black olives (optional)
- Sour cream, salsa, and guacamole for serving

1. Preheat your oven to 350°F.

2. In a large skillet, cook the ground beef over medium heat until browned and crumbled, about 5-7 minutes. Drain any excess fat.

3. Stir in the taco seasoning and water. Simmer for 5 minutes, stirring occasionally, until the sauce has thickened.

4. Spread the tortilla chips out in a single layer on a large baking sheet or oven-safe platter.

5. Spoon the seasoned ground beef evenly over the chips, then top with the shredded cheddar cheese.

6. Bake for 5-7 minutes, or until the cheese is melted and bubbly.

7. Remove the nachos from the oven and top with the drained and rinsed black beans, diced tomatoes, and sliced black olives (if using).

8. Serve the beef nachos immediately, with sour cream, salsa, and guacamole on the side for dipping and topping.

Tips:
- Use mild taco seasoning for a less spicy flavor.
- Customize the toppings to your teen's preferences, such as adding jalapeños or diced onions.
- For a heartier meal, serve the nachos with a side of Mexican rice or a simple salad.

Did you have fun cooking this dish?

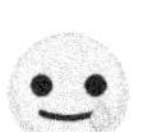 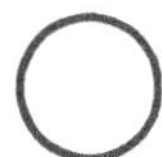 ○    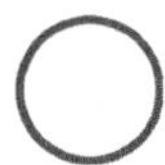 ○

How would you rate this dish?

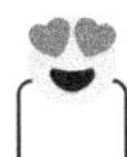 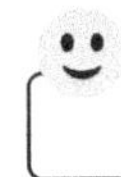   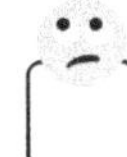 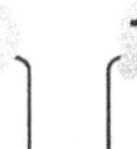 

47. Stuffed crust pizza

 *Let's do that and fill in the time here* 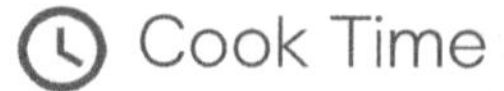 Prep Time :   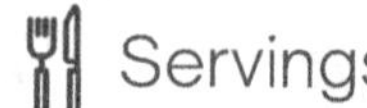 Cook Time :   Servings :

Write 5 friends with whom you want to share this dish

Is this dish easy or difficult for you to make?

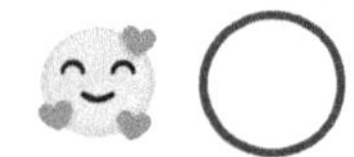

INGREDIENTS

- 1 (13.8 oz) package refrigerated pizza dough
- 8 mozzarella cheese sticks, cut in half
- 1 cup shredded mozzarella cheese
- 1 cup pizza sauce
- Desired pizza toppings (such as pepperoni, mushrooms, bell peppers, etc.)

1. Preheat your oven to 400°F. Grease a 12-inch pizza pan or baking sheet.

2. Roll out the pizza dough into a 12-inch circle on a lightly floured surface.

3. Arrange the 16 pieces of mozzarella cheese stick around the outer edge of the dough, leaving about 1 inch of dough hanging over the edge.

4. Fold the overhanging dough over the cheese sticks, pressing to seal.

5. Transfer the pizza dough to the prepared pan.

6. Spread the pizza sauce evenly over the dough, leaving a 1-inch border.

7. Sprinkle the shredded mozzarella cheese over the sauce.

8. Add your desired pizza toppings on top of the cheese.

9. Bake for 18-22 minutes, or until the crust is golden brown and the cheese is melted and bubbly.

10. Let the pizza cool for 5 minutes before slicing and serving.

Tips:
- Use low-moisture mozzarella cheese sticks for the best texture.
- Customize the toppings to your teen's preferences, such as pepperoni, sausage, vegetables, etc.

Did you have fun cooking this dish?

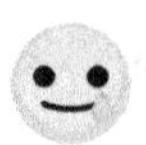  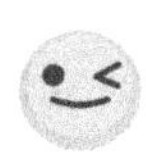 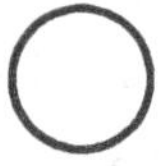

How would you rate this dish?

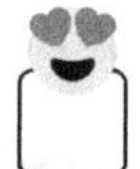 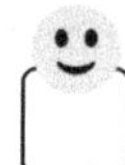 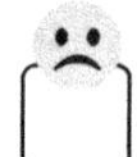 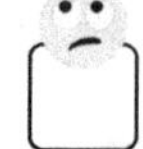 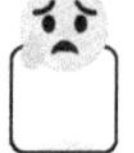

48. Chili cheese fries

Let's do that and fill in the time here    Prep Time :   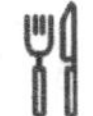 Cook Time :   Servings :

Write 5 friends with whom you want to share this dish
....
....
....
....
....

Is this dish easy or difficult for you to make?

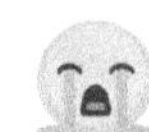 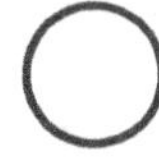 ◯   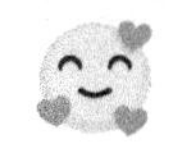 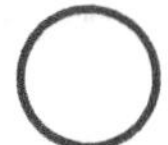 ◯

INGREDIENTS

- 2 lbs russet potatoes, cut into 1/4-inch thick fries
- 2 tablespoons vegetable oil
- 1 lb ground beef
- 1 packet chili seasoning mix
- 1 (15 oz) can tomato sauce
- 1 (15 oz) can kidney beans, drained and rinsed
- 2 cups shredded cheddar cheese
- Sour cream, chopped green onions, and jalapeños (optional toppings)

1. Preheat your oven to 400°F. Line a large baking sheet with parchment paper.

2. Toss the cut fries with the vegetable oil and spread them out in a single layer on the prepared baking sheet.

3. Bake the fries for 20-25 minutes, flipping halfway, until golden brown and crispy.

4. While the fries are baking, cook the ground beef in a skillet over medium heat until browned and crumbled, about 5-7 minutes. Drain any excess fat.

5. Stir in the chili seasoning mix and tomato sauce. Simmer for 5 minutes, then stir in the kidney beans. Reduce heat to low and keep warm.

6. Once the fries are done, remove them from the oven and top with the chili mixture, followed by the shredded cheddar cheese.

7. Return the fries to the oven for an additional 5 minutes, or until the cheese is melted and bubbly.

8. Serve the chili cheese fries immediately, with sour cream, chopped green onions, and jalapeños (if desired) on the side.

Tips:
- Use frozen french fries for a quicker prep time.
- Adjust the amount of chili seasoning to control the spice level.
- Offer additional toppings like diced tomatoes, bacon bits, or guacamole for customization.

Did you have fun cooking this dish?

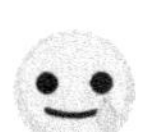 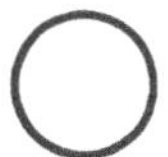 ◯    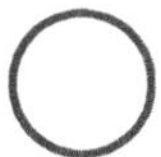 ◯

How would you rate this dish?

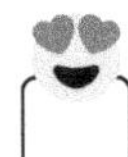 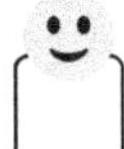 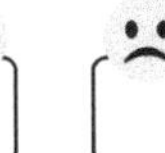  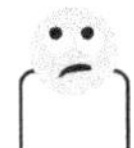 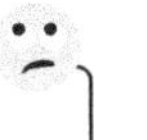 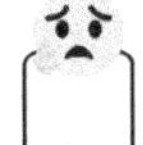 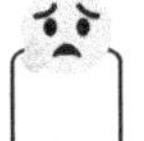

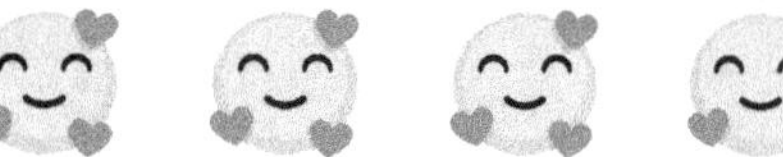

49. Meatball sub

 Prep Time : 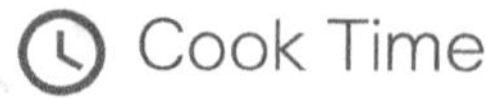 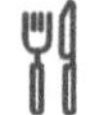 Cook Time : Servings :

Is this dish easy or difficult for you to make?

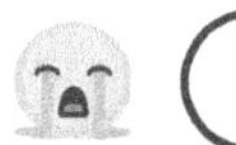 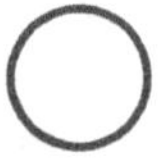 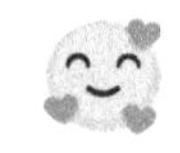 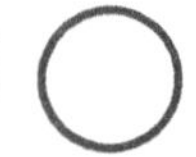

Write 5 friends with whom you want to share this dish

INGREDIENTS

- 1 lb ground beef
- 1/2 cup breadcrumbs
- 1/4 cup grated Parmesan cheese
- 1 egg
- 2 cloves garlic, minced
- 1 teaspoon dried oregano
- 1/2 teaspoon salt
- 1/4 teaspoon black pepper
- 1 (24 oz) jar marinara sauce
- 4 hoagie or sub rolls, split lengthwise
- 8 slices provolone cheese

1. Preheat your oven to 400°F.

2. In a large bowl, combine the ground beef, breadcrumbs, Parmesan cheese, egg, garlic, oregano, salt, and pepper. Mix until well incorporated.

3. Roll the mixture into 12 equal-sized meatballs, about 2 inches in diameter.

4. Place the meatballs on a baking sheet and bake for 15-18 minutes, or until cooked through.

5. In a medium saucepan, heat the marinara sauce over medium heat.

6. Add the cooked meatballs to the sauce and simmer for 5-10 minutes, allowing the flavors to meld.

7. Place the split sub rolls on a baking sheet. Top each roll with 3 meatballs and some of the marinara sauce.

8. Top the meatballs with a slice of provolone cheese.

9. Bake the meatball subs for 5-7 minutes, or until the cheese is melted and bubbly.

10. Serve the meatball subs warm.

Tips:
- Use lean ground beef to keep the meatballs from being too greasy.
- Customize the meatballs by adding other herbs and spices, such as basil, parsley, or red pepper flakes.

Did you have fun cooking this dish?

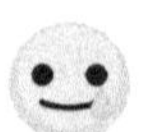 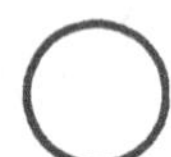  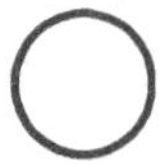

How would you rate this dish?

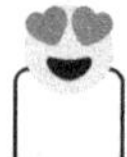 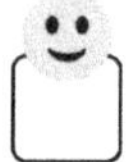  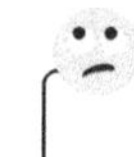 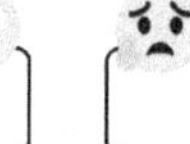 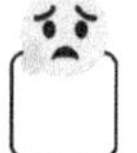

50. Chicken quesadilla

 Prep Time : 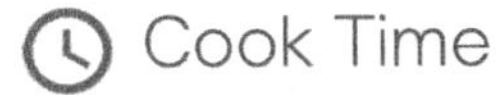 Cook Time : 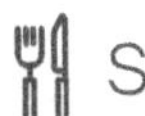 Servings :

Let's do that and fill in the time here

Write 5 friends with whom you want to share this dish

Is this dish easy or difficult for you to make?

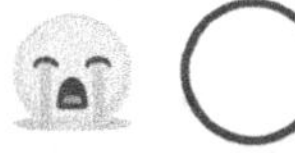 ○ 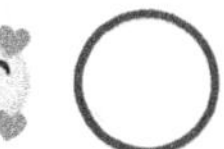 ○

INGREDIENTS

- 1 lb boneless, skinless chicken breasts, cubed
- 1 tablespoon olive oil
- 1 teaspoon chili powder
- 1/2 teaspoon cumin
- 1/4 teaspoon garlic powder
- Salt and pepper to taste
- 8 (8-inch) flour tortillas
- 2 cups shredded cheddar or Monterey Jack cheese
- Salsa, sour cream, and guacamole for serving

1. In a large skillet, heat the olive oil over medium-high heat. Add the cubed chicken and season with the chili powder, cumin, garlic powder, salt, and pepper. Cook, stirring occasionally, until the chicken is cooked through, about 6-8 minutes. Remove from heat and set aside.

2. Lay 4 of the tortillas on a clean work surface. Divide the cooked chicken evenly among the tortillas, spreading it out in an even layer.

3. Sprinkle 1/2 cup of the shredded cheese over the chicken on each tortilla.

4. Top each quesadilla with the remaining 4 tortillas.

5. Heat a large skillet or griddle over medium heat. Working in batches if necessary, cook the quesadillas for 2-3 minutes per side, or until the tortillas are golden brown and the cheese is melted.

6. Remove the quesadillas from the heat and cut each one into 4 triangular wedges.

7. Serve the chicken quesadillas warm, with salsa, sour cream, and guacamole on the side for dipping and topping.

Tips:
- Use a rotisserie chicken or leftover cooked chicken to save time.
- Customize the fillings by adding diced bell peppers, onions, or black beans.
- For a healthier option, use whole wheat tortillas.
- Serve the quesadillas with a side salad or fresh fruit for a balanced meal.

Did you have fun cooking this dish?

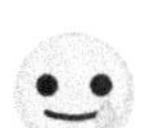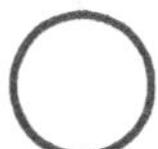 ○  ○

How would you rate this dish?

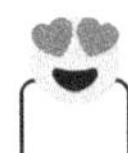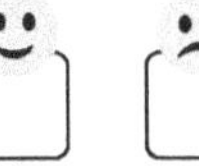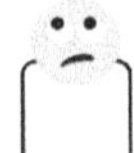

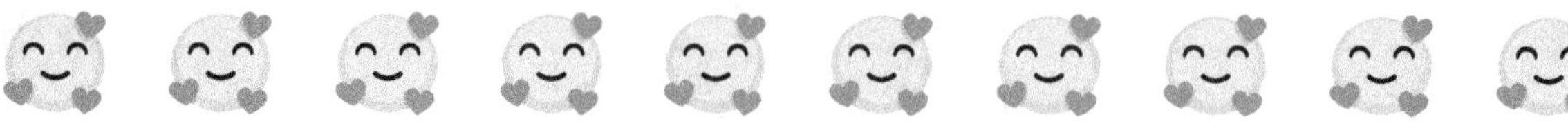

51. Lasagna

 Prep Time : 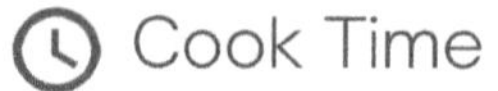 Cook Time :  Servings :

Write 5 friends with whom you want to share this dish

....

....

....

....

....

INGREDIENTS

- 9 lasagna noodles
- 1 lb ground beef
- 1 onion, diced
- 2 cloves garlic, minced
- 1 (24 oz) jar marinara sauce
- 1 (15 oz) can tomato sauce
- 1 teaspoon dried oregano
- 1/2 teaspoon dried basil
- 1/4 teaspoon red pepper flakes (optional)
- 1 (15 oz) container ricotta cheese
- 2 cups shredded mozzarella cheese
- 1/2 cup grated Parmesan cheese
- 1 egg
- Salt and pepper to taste

Is this dish easy or difficult for you to make?

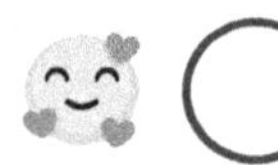

1. Preheat your oven to 375°F.

2. Bring a large pot of salted water to a boil. Cook the lasagna noodles according to package instructions until al dente. Drain and set aside.

3. In a large skillet, cook the ground beef over medium heat until browned and crumbled, 5-7 minutes. Drain any excess fat.

4. Add the diced onion and minced garlic to the skillet. Cook for 2-3 minutes until the onion is translucent.

5. Stir in the marinara sauce, tomato sauce, oregano, basil, and red pepper flakes (if using). Simmer for 10 minutes, then remove from heat.

6. In a medium bowl, mix together the ricotta cheese, 1 cup of the mozzarella cheese, the Parmesan cheese, and the egg. Season with salt and pepper.

7. Spread 1 cup of the meat sauce in the bottom of a 9x13 inch baking dish.

8. Layer 3 lasagna noodles over the sauce. Spread half of the ricotta cheese mixture over the noodles, then top with 1 cup of the meat sauce.

9. Repeat the noodle, ricotta, and sauce layers. Top with the remaining 3 lasagna noodles and the remaining meat sauce.

10. Sprinkle the remaining 1 cup of mozzarella cheese over the top. Cover the dish with aluminum foil and bake for 30 minutes.

Did you have fun cooking this dish?

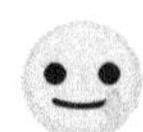  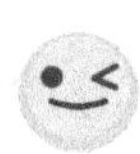 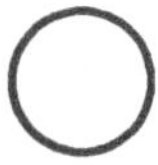

How would you rate this dish?

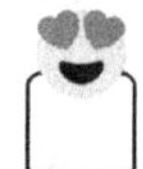 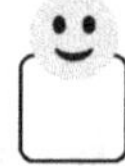  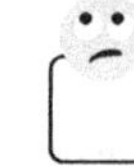 

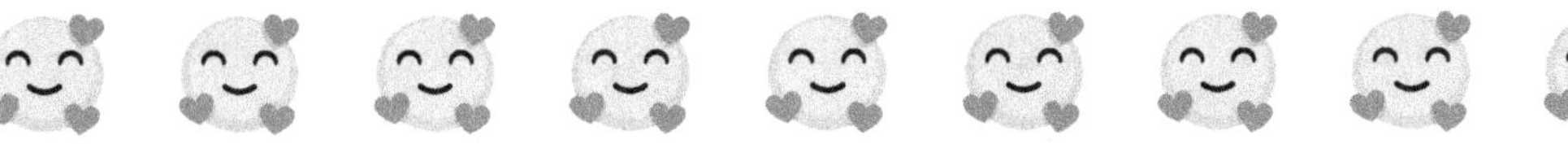

52. Cheesy garlic bread

 Prep Time :    Cook Time :   Servings :

Write 5 friends with whom you want to share this dish

....
....
....
....
....

Is this dish easy or difficult for you to make?

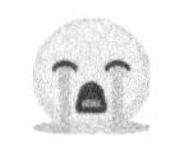 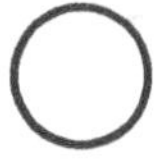 ◯   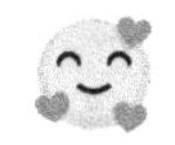 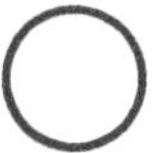 ◯

INGREDIENTS

- 1 loaf of French or Italian bread, cut in half lengthwise
- 1/2 cup (1 stick) unsalted butter, softened
- 3 cloves garlic, minced
- 1 teaspoon dried parsley
- 1/4 teaspoon salt
- 1 1/2 cups shredded mozzarella cheese
- 1/4 cup grated Parmesan cheese

1. Preheat your oven to 400°F. Line a baking sheet with parchment paper.

2. In a small bowl, mix together the softened butter, minced garlic, dried parsley, and salt until well combined.

3. Place the halved bread loaf, cut-side up, on the prepared baking sheet.

4. Spread the garlic butter mixture evenly over the cut surfaces of the bread.

5. Sprinkle the shredded mozzarella cheese and grated Parmesan cheese over the top of the bread.

6. Bake for 10-12 minutes, or until the cheese is melted and bubbly.

7. Remove the cheesy garlic bread from the oven and let it cool for 2-3 minutes.

8. Slice the bread into individual pieces and serve warm.

Tips:
- Use a crusty French or Italian bread for the best texture.
- Adjust the amount of garlic to your teen's preference.
- For extra flavor, add a pinch of dried oregano or basil to the butter mixture.
- Serve the cheesy garlic bread as a side dish or appetizer.

Did you have fun cooking this dish?

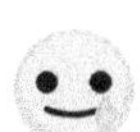 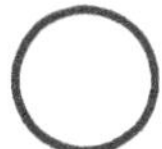 ◯    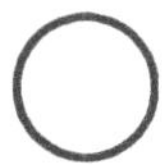 ◯

How would you rate this dish?

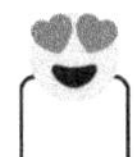 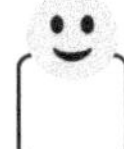 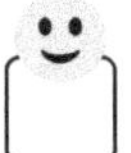  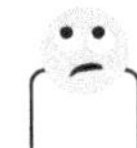 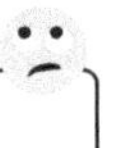 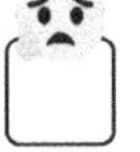

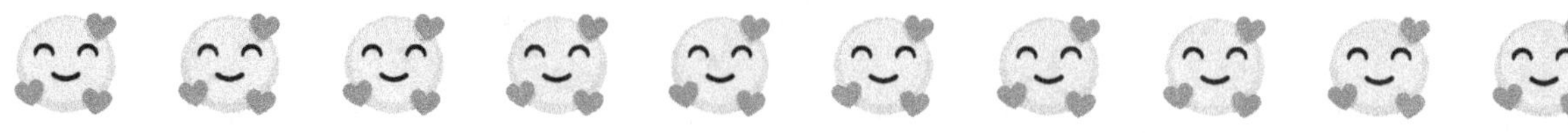

53. Chicken wings (various flavors)

 Prep Time :   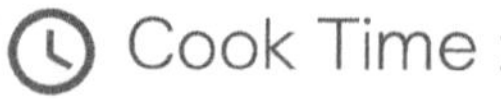 Cook Time :   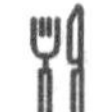 Servings :

Write 5 friends with whom you want to share this dish

....
....
....
....
....

Is this dish easy or difficult for you to make?

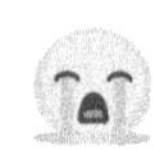 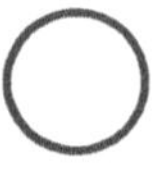 ◯    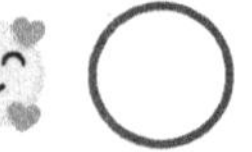 ◯

INGREDIENTS

- 2 lbs chicken wings, drumettes and flats separated
- 2 tablespoons olive oil
- 1 teaspoon garlic powder
- 1 teaspoon paprika
- 1/2 teaspoon salt
- 1/4 teaspoon black pepper

Ingredients:
- 2 lbs chicken wings
- 1/2 cup hot sauce (like Frank's RedHot)
- 1/3 cup butter
- Salt and pepper to taste

Instructions:
1. Preheat oven to 400°F (200°C).
2. Season wings with salt and pepper.
3. Bake for 45-50 minutes, turning halfway through.
4. Melt butter and mix with hot sauce.
5. Toss cooked wings in sauce.

2. Honey Garlic Wings:

Ingredients:
- 2 lbs chicken wings
- 1/3 cup honey
- 1/4 cup soy sauce
- 4 cloves garlic, minced
- 2 tbsp vegetable oil
- Salt and pepper to taste

Instructions:
1. Mix honey, soy sauce, garlic, and oil.
2. Marinate wings for 2 hours.
3. Preheat oven to 375°F (190°C).
4. Bake for 45 minutes, turning halfway.
5. Brush with remaining marinade before serving.

Did you have fun cooking this dish?

  ◯    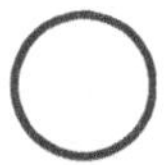 ◯

How would you rate this dish?

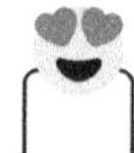 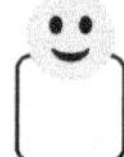 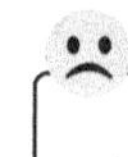 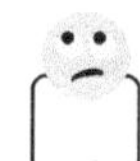 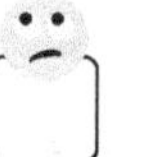 

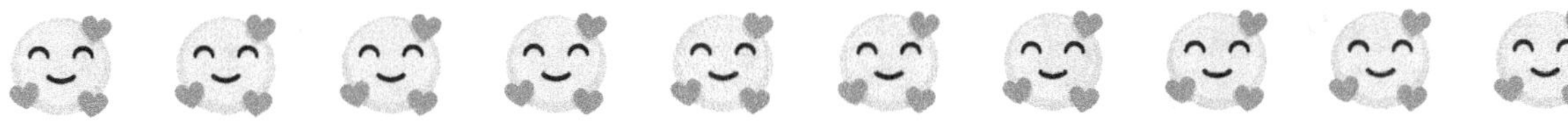

54. Bacon mac and cheese

Prep Time : 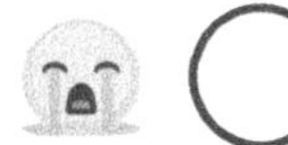

Cook Time : 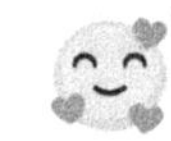

Servings : 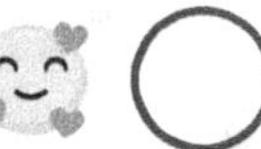

Write 5 friends with whom you want to share this dish

....

....

....

....

Is this dish easy or difficult for you to make?

 ◯   ◯

INGREDIENTS

- 8 oz elbow macaroni
- 4 slices bacon, diced
- 2 tablespoons unsalted butter
- 2 tablespoons all-purpose flour
- 2 cups milk
- 1 1/2 cups shredded cheddar cheese
- 1/2 cup grated Parmesan cheese
- 1/4 teaspoon salt
- 1/4 teaspoon black pepper

1. Bring a large pot of salted water to a boil. Cook the elbow macaroni according to package instructions until al dente. Drain and set aside.

2. In a large skillet, cook the diced bacon over medium heat until crispy, about 5-7 minutes. Transfer the cooked bacon to a paper towel-lined plate and set aside.

3. In the same skillet, melt the butter over medium heat. Whisk in the flour and cook for 1 minute, stirring constantly.

4. Gradually whisk in the milk and bring the mixture to a simmer. Cook, stirring frequently, until the sauce has thickened, about 5 minutes.

5. Remove the skillet from the heat and stir in the shredded cheddar cheese, Parmesan cheese, salt, and black pepper until the cheese is melted and the sauce is smooth.

6. Add the cooked macaroni to the cheese sauce and stir to combine.

7. Fold in the cooked bacon pieces. Serve the bacon mac and cheese warm.

Tips:
- Use a combination of different cheeses, such as cheddar, Monterey Jack, or Gruyère, for more flavor.
- For a crunchy topping, sprinkle some panko breadcrumbs over the mac and cheese before baking.
- Serve the bacon mac and cheese with a side salad or steamed broccoli for a balanced meal.

Did you have fun cooking this dish?

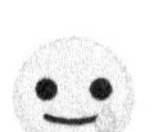 ◯    ◯

How would you rate this dish?

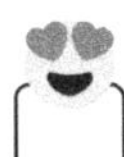 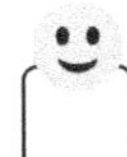   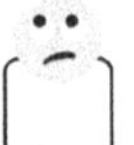

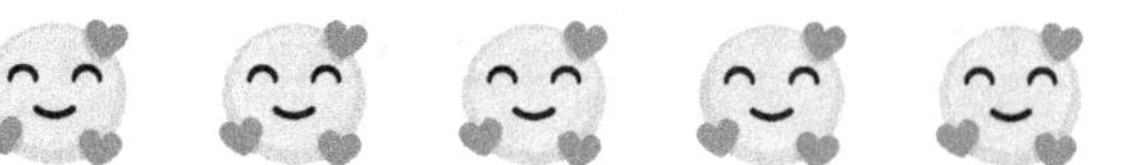

55. Pizza bagels

Let's do that and fill in the time here  Prep Time :   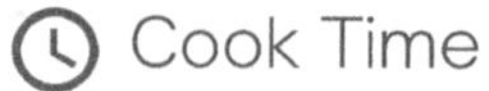 Cook Time :   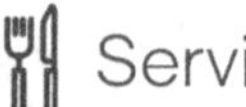 Servings :

Write 5 friends with whom you want to share this dish
....
....
....
....
....

Is this dish easy or difficult for you to make?

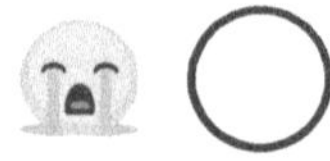 ◯   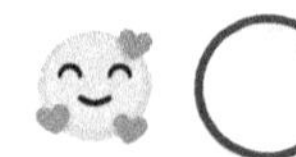 ◯

INGREDIENTS

- 4 plain bagels, split in half
- 1 cup marinara or pizza sauce
- 1 cup shredded mozzarella cheese
- Pepperoni slices (optional)
- Other desired toppings (such as mushrooms, bell peppers, olives, etc.)

1. Preheat your oven to 400°F. Line a baking sheet with parchment paper.

2. Place the split bagel halves on the prepared baking sheet.

3. Spread about 2-3 tablespoons of marinara or pizza sauce evenly over each bagel half.

4. Sprinkle the shredded mozzarella cheese over the sauce, covering the bagels completely.

5. If using, arrange the pepperoni slices or other desired toppings on top of the cheese.

6. Bake the pizza bagels for 8-10 minutes, or until the cheese is melted and bubbly.

7. Remove the pizza bagels from the oven and let them cool for 2-3 minutes before serving.

Tips:
- Use mini bagels or English muffins for a smaller, kid-friendly size.
- Encourage your teen to customize their pizza bagels with their favorite toppings.
- Serve the pizza bagels with a side salad or fresh fruit for a balanced meal.
- For a healthier option, use whole wheat or multigrain bagels.

Did you have fun cooking this dish?

 ◯    ◯

How would you rate this dish?

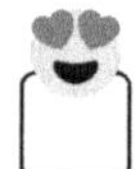 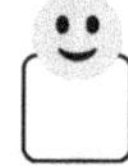   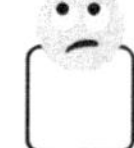 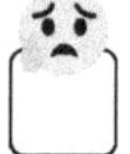

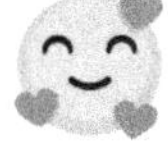 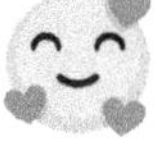 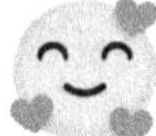 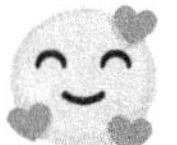 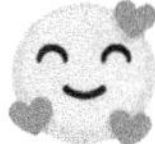 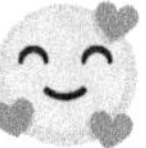 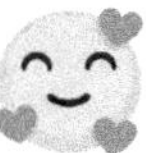 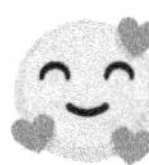 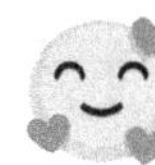 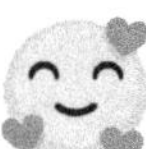

56. Loaded nachos

Let's do that and fill in the time here  Prep Time :   Cook Time :   Servings :

Write 5 friends with whom you want to share this dish

....
....
....
....
....

INGREDIENTS

- 1 bag (13 oz) tortilla chips
- 1 lb ground beef
- 1 packet taco seasoning
- 1/2 cup water
- 1 (15 oz) can black beans, drained and rinsed
- 1 cup shredded cheddar cheese
- 1 cup shredded Monterey Jack cheese
- 1 cup diced tomatoes
- 1/2 cup sliced black olives (optional)
- Sour cream, salsa, and guacamole for serving

Did you have fun cooking this dish?

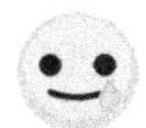 ◯    ◯

How would you rate this dish?

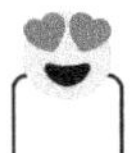 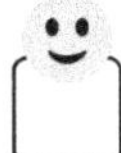 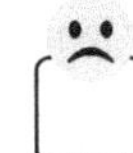 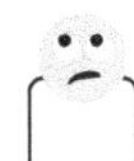 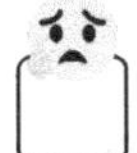

Is this dish easy or difficult for you to make?

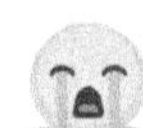 ◯   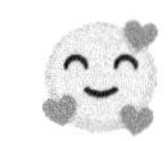 ◯

1. Preheat your oven to 350°F.

2. In a large skillet, cook the ground beef over medium heat until browned and crumbled, about 5-7 minutes. Drain any excess fat.

3. Stir in the taco seasoning and water. Simmer for 5 minutes, until the sauce has thickened.

4. Spread the tortilla chips out in a single layer on a large baking sheet or oven-safe platter.

5. Spoon the seasoned ground beef evenly over the chips, then top with the drained and rinsed black beans.

6. Sprinkle the shredded cheddar and Monterey Jack cheeses over the top.

7. Bake for 5-7 minutes, or until the cheese is melted and bubbly.

8. Remove the nachos from the oven and top with the diced tomatoes and sliced black olives (if using).

9. Serve the loaded nachos immediately, with sour cream, salsa, and guacamole on the side for dipping and topping.

Tips:
- Use mild taco seasoning for a less spicy flavor.
- Customize the toppings to your teen's preferences, such as adding jalapeños, corn, or scallions.
- For a heartier meal, serve the nachos with a side of Mexican rice or a simple salad.

 Prep Time : 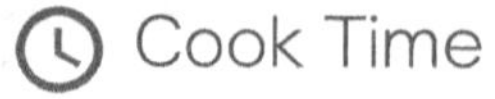  Cook Time : Servings :

Let's do that and fill in the time here

Write 5 friends with whom you want to share this dish

Is this dish easy or difficult for you to make?

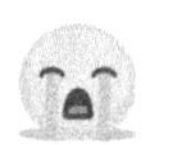 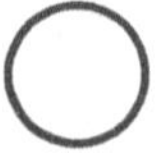 ⭕ 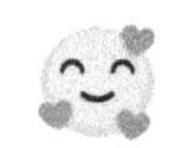  ⭕

INGREDIENTS

- 1 lb ground beef
- 1 packet taco seasoning
- 1/2 cup water
- 12 taco shells or soft tortillas
- 1 cup shredded lettuce
- 1 cup diced tomatoes
- 1 cup shredded cheddar or Mexican blend cheese
- Sour cream, salsa, and other desired toppings

1. In a large skillet, cook the ground beef over medium heat until browned and crumbled, 5-7 minutes. Drain any excess fat.

2. Stir in the taco seasoning and water. Simmer for 5 minutes, stirring occasionally, until the sauce has thickened.

3. Warm the taco shells or tortillas according to package instructions.

4. To assemble the tacos, place a spoonful of the seasoned ground beef into each taco shell or tortilla.

5. Top the beef with shredded lettuce, diced tomatoes, and shredded cheese.

6. Serve the beef tacos with sour cream, salsa, and any other desired toppings on the side.

Tips:
- Use mild taco seasoning for a less spicy flavor.
- Customize the toppings to your preferences, such as adding diced onions, jalapeños, or guacamole.
- For a healthier option, use whole wheat tortillas or lettuce wraps instead of taco shells.
- Serve the beef tacos with a side of Mexican rice or refried beans for a more complete meal.

Did you have fun cooking this dish?

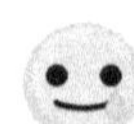 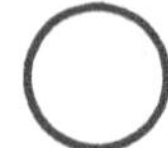 ⭕ 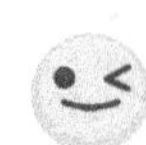 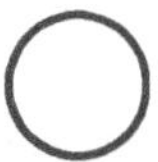 ⭕

How would you rate this dish?

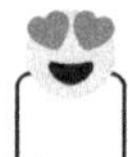 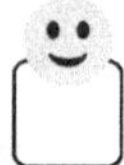 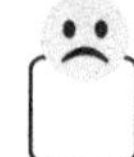 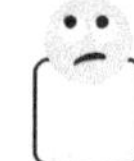 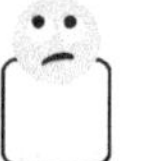 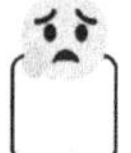

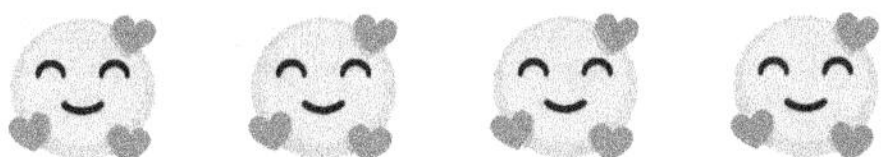

58. Chicken burrito

 Prep Time :　 Cook Time :　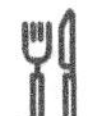 Servings :

Write 5 friends with whom you want to share this dish

....

....

....

....

....

INGREDIENTS

- 1 lb boneless, skinless chicken breasts
- 1 packet taco seasoning
- 1/2 cup water
- 1 (15 oz) can black beans, drained and rinsed
- 1 cup cooked rice
- 1 cup shredded cheddar or Monterey Jack cheese
- 8 large flour tortillas
- Salsa, sour cream, and guacamole for serving

Is this dish easy or difficult for you to make?

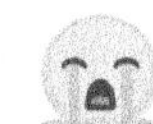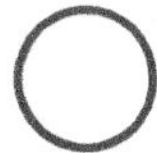 ○　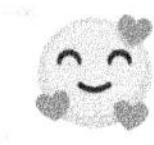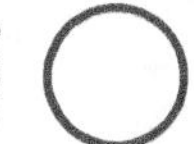 ○

1. In a large skillet, cook the chicken over medium heat until no longer pink, about 6-8 minutes. Shred or chop the cooked chicken into bite-sized pieces.

2. Add the taco seasoning and water to the skillet with the chicken. Stir to combine and simmer for 5 minutes, until the sauce has thickened.

3. Warm the tortillas according to package instructions to make them pliable.

4. Lay a tortilla flat and layer with 2-3 tablespoons of the seasoned chicken, 2-3 tablespoons of black beans, 2-3 tablespoons of cooked rice, and 2-3 tablespoons of shredded cheese.

5. Fold the bottom of the tortilla up over the filling, then fold in the sides and continue rolling up tightly into a burrito shape.

6. Place the burrito seam-side down on a plate. Repeat with the remaining tortillas and fillings.

7. Serve the chicken burritos warm, with salsa, sour cream, and guacamole on the side for topping and dipping.

Tips:
- Use mild taco seasoning for a less spicy flavor.
- Customize the fillings to your teen's preferences, such as adding diced tomatoes, lettuce, or corn.
- Wrap individual burritos in foil to keep them warm and portable.

Did you have fun cooking this dish?

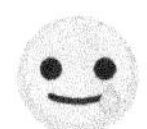 ○　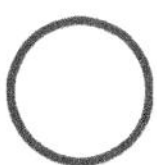 ○

How would you rate this dish?

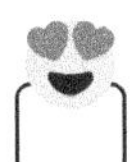  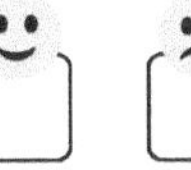 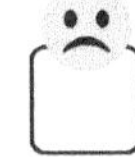 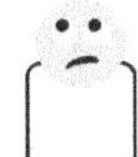 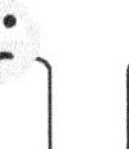 

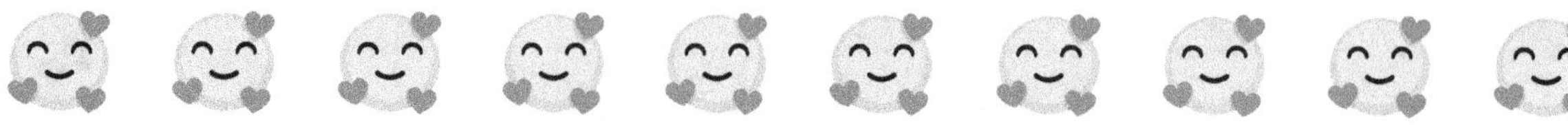

59. Cheese stuffed breadsticks

 *Let's do that and fill in the time here* Prep Time :   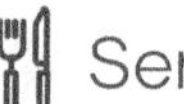 Cook Time :   Servings :

Write 5 friends with whom you want to share this dish

....

....

....

....

....

INGREDIENTS

- 1 lb pizza dough, store-bought or homemade
- 8 oz mozzarella cheese, cut into 1-inch cubes
- 2 tbsp butter, melted
- 1 tsp garlic powder
- 1 tsp Italian seasoning
- 1/4 cup grated Parmesan cheese

Is this dish easy or difficult for you to make?

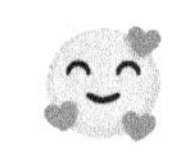 ◯   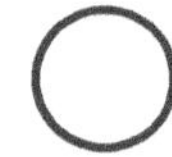 ◯

1. Preheat your oven to 400°F. Line a baking sheet with parchment paper.

2. Divide the pizza dough into 12 equal pieces. Take one piece and flatten it into a rectangle. Place a cube of mozzarella cheese in the center, then wrap the dough around the cheese, pinching the seams to seal.

3. Place the stuffed breadstick seam-side down on the prepared baking sheet. Repeat with the remaining dough and cheese cubes.

4. In a small bowl, mix together the melted butter, garlic powder, and Italian seasoning. Brush this mixture over the top of the stuffed breadsticks.

5. Sprinkle the grated Parmesan cheese over the top of the breadsticks.

6. Bake for 15-18 minutes, until the breadsticks are golden brown.

7. Serve the warm, cheesy breadsticks with marinara sauce for dipping, if desired.

These cheese stuffed breadsticks are fun, easy to eat, and full of melty, gooey cheese - perfect for young teens! The garlic and Italian seasoning add great flavor too.

Did you have fun cooking this dish?

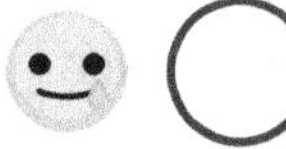 ◯   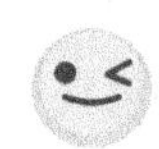 ◯

How would you rate this dish?

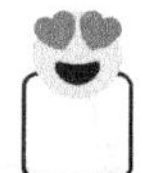 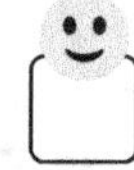 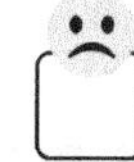 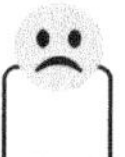 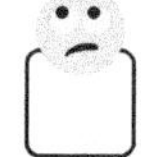 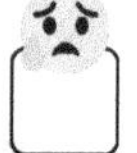

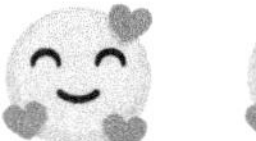 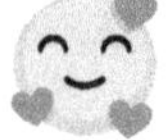 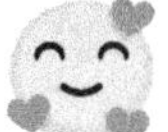 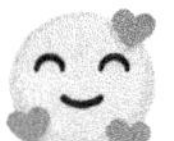 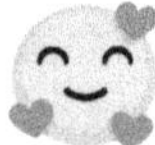 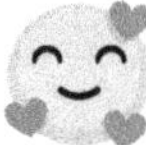 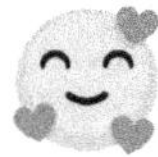 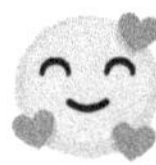 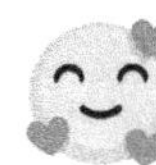 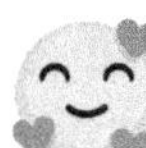

60. Mini corn dogs

Let's do that and fill in the time here ⊘ Prep Time :   ○ Cook Time :   🍴 Servings :

Write 5 friends with whom you want to share this dish
....
....
....
....
....

Is this dish easy or difficult for you to make?

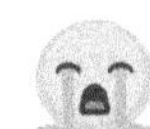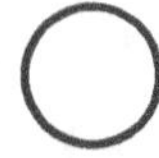 ○   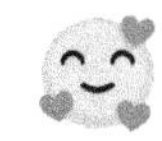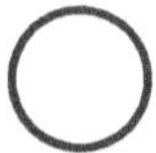 ○

INGREDIENTS

- 1 cup all-purpose flour
- 1/2 cup yellow cornmeal
- 1 tbsp white sugar
- 1 tsp baking powder
- 1/2 tsp salt
- 1 egg
- 3/4 cup milk
- 1 tbsp vegetable oil
- 12 hot dog mini links or cocktail franks
- Vegetable oil for frying

1. In a medium bowl, whisk together the flour, cornmeal, sugar, baking powder, and salt.

2. In a separate bowl, beat the egg. Then stir in the milk and 1 tbsp of vegetable oil.

3. Pour the wet ingredients into the dry ingredients and stir just until combined (do not overmix).

4. Insert a wooden skewer or toothpick into each mini hot dog.

5. Heat 2-3 inches of vegetable oil in a heavy bottomed pot or Dutch oven to 350°F.

6. Working in batches, dip the skewered hot dogs into the corn dog batter, coating them completely.

7. Carefully lower the battered hot dogs into the hot oil and fry for 2-3 minutes, turning occasionally, until golden brown.

8. Remove the mini corn dogs from the oil using a slotted spoon and place them on a paper towel-lined plate to drain.

9. Serve the mini corn dogs warm, with your favorite dipping sauces like mustard, ketchup, or ranch.

These bite-sized corn dogs are perfect for young teens - they're fun, portable, and easy to eat. The cornmeal batter gives them a delicious crispy exterior.

Did you have fun cooking this dish?

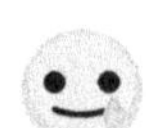 ○    ○

How would you rate this dish?

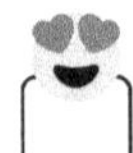 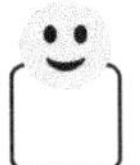 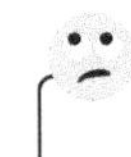 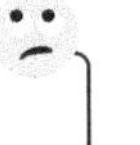 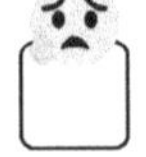

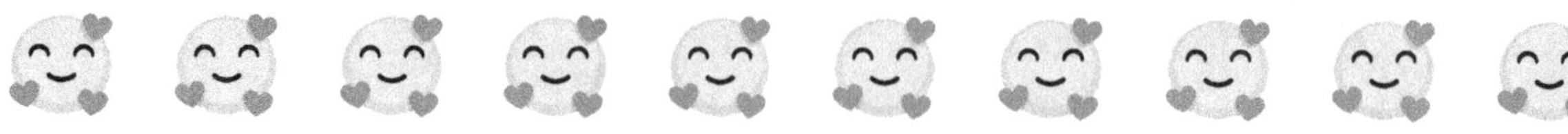

61. BBQ pulled pork sandwich

 *Let's do that and fill in the time here* 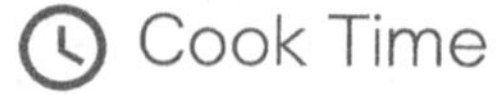 Prep Time :  Cook Time : Servings :

Write 5 friends with whom you want to share this dish

....
....
....
....
....

INGREDIENTS

- 3-4 lb pork shoulder or butt, trimmed of excess fat
- 1 tbsp brown sugar
- 2 tsp smoked paprika
- 1 tsp garlic powder
- 1 tsp onion powder
- 1 tsp salt
- 1/2 tsp black pepper
- 1 cup barbecue sauce (your favorite brand or homemade)
- 8-10 hamburger buns or rolls

Is this dish easy or difficult for you to make?

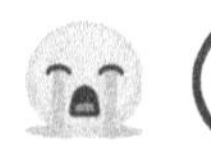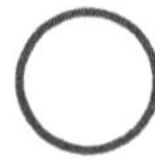 ○   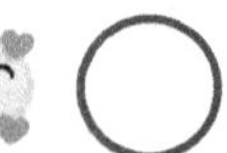 ○

1. In a small bowl, mix together the brown sugar, smoked paprika, garlic powder, onion powder, salt, and black pepper. Rub this seasoning mixture all over the pork.

2. Place the seasoned pork in a slow cooker and cook on low for 8-10 hours, until the meat is very tender and shreds easily with two forks.

3. Remove the pork from the slow cooker and shred it using two forks. Discard any large pieces of fat.

4. Return the shredded pork to the slow cooker and stir in the barbecue sauce. Let it heat through, about 15-20 minutes.

5. Serve the BBQ pulled pork on the hamburger buns or rolls. Top with coleslaw, pickles, or other desired toppings.

Enjoy your delicious BBQ pulled pork sandwiches! The slow cooking makes the pork incredibly tender and flavorful.

Did you have fun cooking this dish?

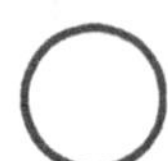 ○   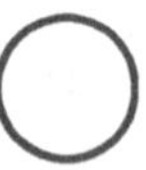 ○

How would you rate this dish?

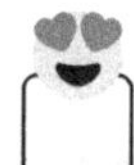 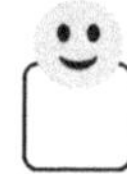  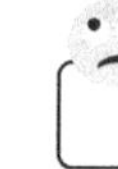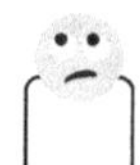 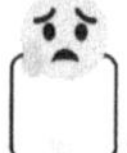

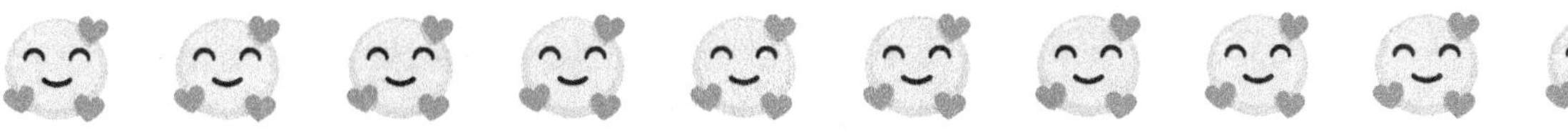

62. Chicken bacon ranch wrap

Let's do that and fill in the time here

 Prep Time : 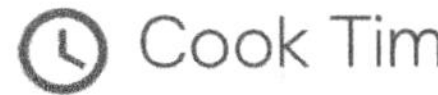  Cook Time : Servings :

Write 5 friends with whom you want to share this dish

....
....
....
....
....

Is this dish easy or difficult for you to make?

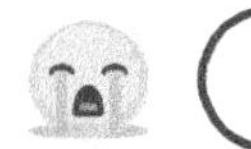 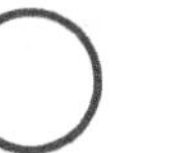 ◯   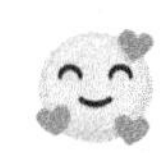 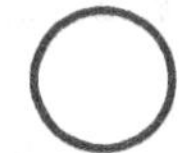 ◯

INGREDIENTS

- 4 large flour tortillas or wraps
- 2 cups cooked, shredded chicken
- 6 slices bacon, cooked and crumbled
- 1 cup shredded cheddar cheese
- 1/2 cup ranch dressing
- 1/4 cup diced tomatoes
- 1/4 cup shredded lettuce

1. In a medium bowl, mix together the shredded chicken, crumbled bacon, cheddar cheese, and ranch dressing until well combined.

2. Lay the tortillas or wraps out flat on a clean surface. Divide the chicken mixture evenly among the 4 wraps, placing it in the center.

3. Top each wrap with some diced tomatoes and shredded lettuce.

4. Fold the bottom of the wrap up over the filling, then fold in the sides and continue rolling it up tightly into a burrito shape.

5. If desired, you can wrap the wraps in foil or parchment paper to help them hold their shape.

6. Serve the chicken bacon ranch wraps immediately, or refrigerate until ready to eat.

These wraps are perfect for young teens because they're portable, easy to eat, and full of flavor. The combination of chicken, bacon, cheese, and ranch is always a hit. You can also customize the fillings to your teen's preferences.

Did you have fun cooking this dish?

 ◯    ◯

How would you rate this dish?

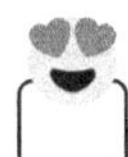 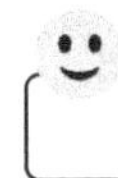 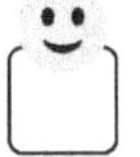 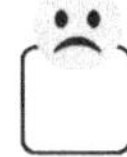 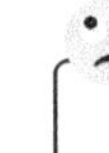 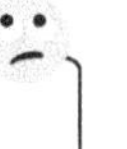 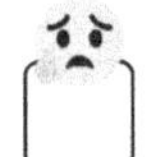

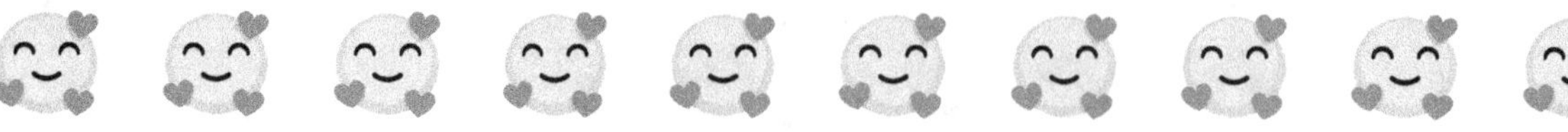

63. Loaded potato skins

  Prep Time : 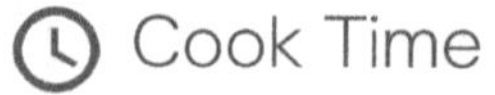  Cook Time : Servings :

Write 5 friends with whom you want to share this dish

Is this dish easy or difficult for you to make?

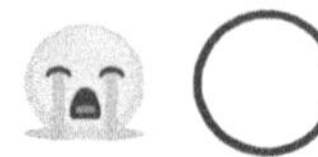 ◯  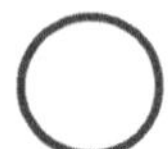 ◯

INGREDIENTS

- 4 medium russet potatoes
- 2 tbsp olive oil
- 1/2 tsp salt
- 1/4 tsp black pepper
- 1 cup shredded cheddar cheese
- 4 slices bacon, cooked and crumbled
- 2 green onions, sliced
- Sour cream for serving (optional)

1. Preheat your oven to 400°F. Wash the potatoes and prick them several times with a fork.

2. Bake the potatoes directly on the oven rack for 50-60 minutes, until they are tender when squeezed. Allow to cool slightly.

3. Cut the potatoes in half lengthwise. Scoop out the insides, leaving about 1/4 inch of potato flesh attached to the skin.

4. Brush the potato skins with the olive oil and season with salt and pepper.

5. Place the potato skins back on the baking sheet, skin-side up. Bake for 10 minutes.

6. Flip the potato skins over and bake for another 10 minutes, until crispy.

7. Remove the potato skins from the oven and top each one with some shredded cheddar cheese, crumbled bacon, and sliced green onions.

8. Return the loaded potato skins to the oven for 5 more minutes, until the cheese is melted.

9. Serve the loaded potato skins warm, with sour cream on the side if desired.

These loaded potato skins are a fun, shareable snack that young teens will love. The crispy potato skins, melty cheese, and bacon make them irresistible!

Did you have fun cooking this dish?

 ◯ 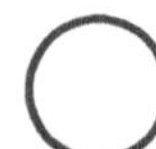  ◯ 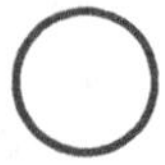

How would you rate this dish?

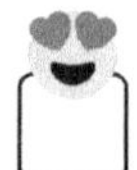 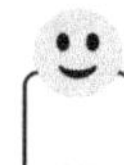  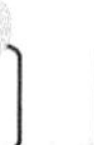 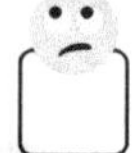 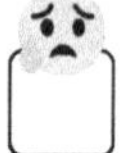

64. Beef and bean burrito

Let's do that and fill in the time here  Prep Time :    Cook Time :   Servings :

Write 5 friends with whom you want to share this dish
....
....
....
....
....

INGREDIENTS

- 1 lb ground beef
- 1 packet taco seasoning
- 1 (15 oz) can black beans, drained and rinsed
- 1 cup cooked rice
- 1 cup shredded cheddar cheese
- 8 large flour tortillas
- Toppings (optional): salsa, sour cream, diced tomatoes, shredded lettuce

Did you have fun cooking this dish?

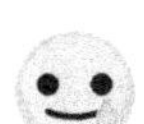 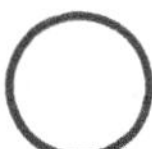 ◯    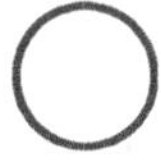 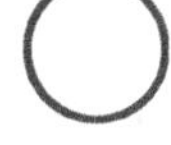 ◯

How would you rate this dish?

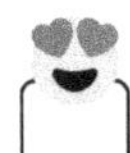 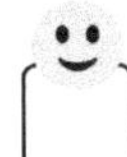 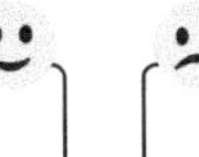  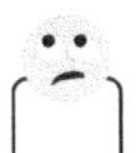 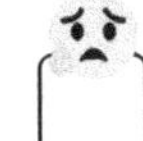 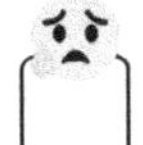

Is this dish easy or difficult for you to make?

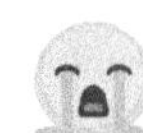 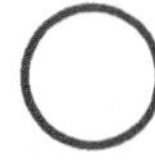 ◯   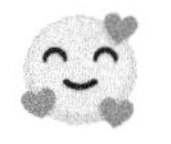 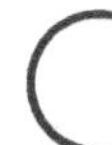 ◯

1. In a large skillet, cook the ground beef over medium heat until browned and crumbled, 5-7 minutes. Drain any excess fat.

2. Stir in the taco seasoning and 1/2 cup of water. Simmer for 5 minutes, until the sauce has thickened.

3. Add the black beans and cooked rice to the beef mixture. Stir to combine.

4. Lay the flour tortillas out on a clean surface. Spoon about 1/2 cup of the beef and bean mixture onto the center of each tortilla.

5. Top each burrito with 2-3 tablespoons of shredded cheddar cheese.

6. Fold the bottom of the tortilla up over the filling, then fold in the sides and continue rolling it up tightly into a burrito shape.

7. Place the burritos seam-side down on a baking sheet.

8. Bake at 350°F for 10-15 minutes, until heated through.

9. Serve the beef and bean burritos warm, with desired toppings on the side.

These hearty burritos are perfect for hungry young teens. The combination of seasoned ground beef, beans, rice, and melty cheese is always a hit. Plus, they're easy to customize with their favorite toppings.

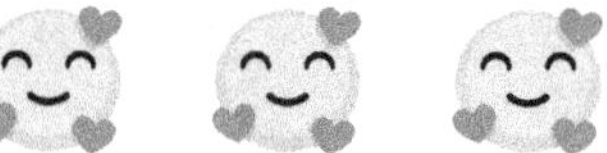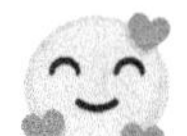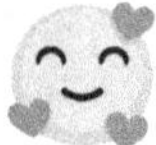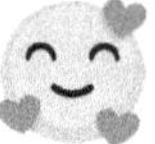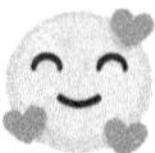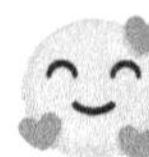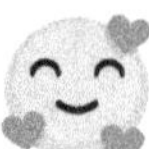

65. Fried mozzarella

Let's do that and fill in the time here

🕐 Prep Time : 🕐 Cook Time : 🍴 Servings :

Write 5 friends with whom you want to share this dish
....
....
....
....
....

INGREDIENTS

- 8 oz block of mozzarella cheese, cut into 1/2-inch thick slices
- 1 cup all-purpose flour
- 2 eggs, beaten
- 1 cup panko breadcrumbs
- 1/2 cup grated Parmesan cheese
- 1 teaspoon dried oregano
- 1/2 teaspoon garlic powder
- 1/4 teaspoon salt
- Vegetable oil for frying
- Marinara sauce for dipping

Is this dish easy or difficult for you to make?

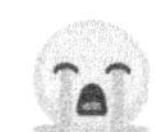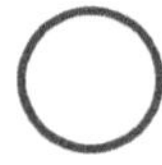 ○   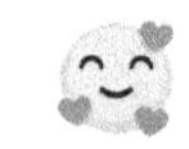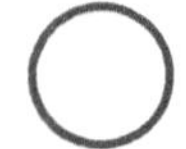 ○

1. Set up a breading station with three shallow dishes:
   - In the first dish, place the all-purpose flour.
   - In the second dish, place the beaten eggs.
   - In the third dish, mix together the panko breadcrumbs, Parmesan cheese, oregano, garlic powder, and salt.

2. Dredge the mozzarella cheese slices in the flour, dip them in the beaten egg, and then coat them in the breadcrumb mixture, pressing gently to help the crumbs adhere.

3. In a large skillet or Dutch oven, heat 1-2 inches of vegetable oil to 350°F.

4. Working in batches, carefully add the breaded mozzarella slices to the hot oil and fry for 2-3 minutes per side, or until golden brown.

5. Transfer the fried mozzarella to a paper towel-lined plate to drain any excess oil.

6. Serve the fried mozzarella warm, with marinara sauce for dipping.

Tips:
- Use low-moisture mozzarella cheese for best results.
- Chill the breaded mozzarella slices for 30 minutes before frying to help them hold their shape.
- For extra crispiness, spray the breaded mozzarella lightly with cooking spray before frying.
- Adjust the frying time as needed, depending on the thickness of your mozzarella slices.

Did you have fun cooking this dish?

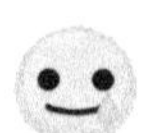 ○   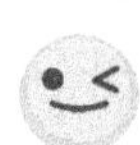 ○

How would you rate this dish?

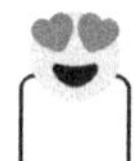 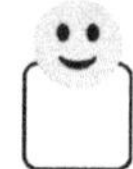 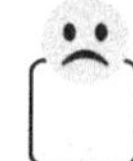 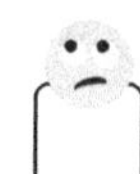 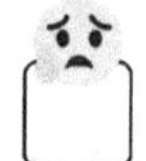

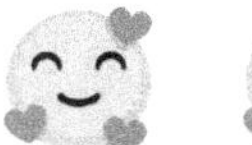 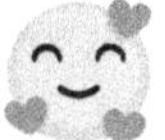 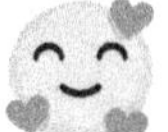 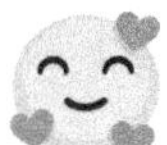 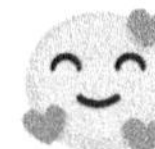 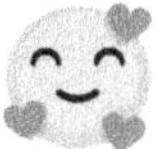 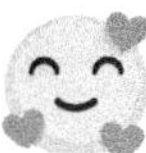   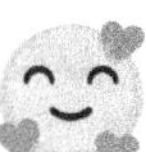

66. Chicken fingers

Let's do that and fill in the time here

Prep Time :

Cook Time :

Servings :

Write 5 friends with whom you want to share this dish

Is this dish easy or difficult for you to make?

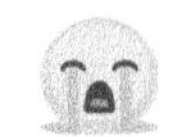 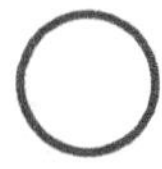 ○     ○

INGREDIENTS

- 1 lb boneless, skinless chicken breasts, cut into strips
- 1 cup all-purpose flour
- 2 eggs, beaten
- 1 cup panko breadcrumbs
- 1 tsp garlic powder
- 1 tsp paprika
- 1/2 tsp salt
- 1/4 tsp black pepper
- Vegetable oil for frying

Dipping Sauces (optional):
- Ranch dressing
- Honey mustard
- BBQ sauce

1. Set up a breading station with three shallow dishes: one with the flour, one with the beaten eggs, and one with the panko breadcrumbs mixed with the garlic powder, paprika, salt, and pepper.

2. Dredge the chicken strips in the flour first, dip them in the egg, and then coat them in the seasoned breadcrumbs, pressing to adhere.

3. In a large skillet or Dutch oven, heat 1-2 inches of vegetable oil to 350°F.

4. Working in batches, carefully add the breaded chicken fingers to the hot oil and fry for 2-3 minutes per side, until golden brown and cooked through.

5. Transfer the fried chicken fingers to a paper towel-lined plate to drain any excess oil.

6. Serve the chicken fingers warm, with your choice of dipping sauces on the side.

These homemade chicken fingers are perfect for young teens - they're crispy, flavorful, and fun to eat. The panko breadcrumbs give them an extra crunchy texture. Offer a variety of dipping sauces so they can customize them to their tastes.

Did you have fun cooking this dish?

  ○    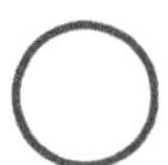 ○

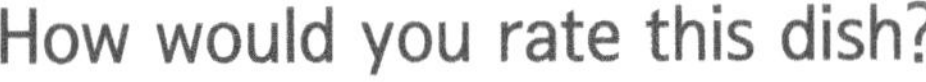

How would you rate this dish?

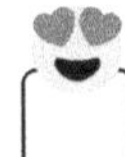 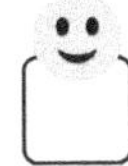   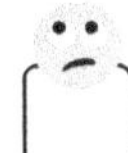 

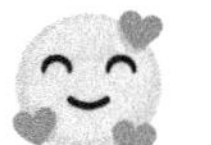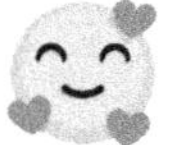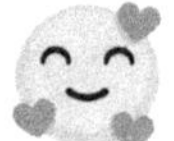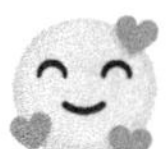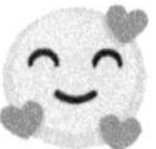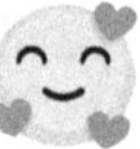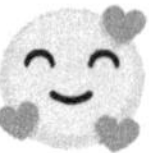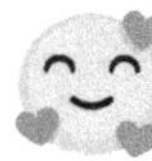

67. Cheese fondue

Let's do that and fill in the time here  Prep Time :   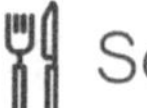 Cook Time :   Servings :

Write 5 friends with whom you want to share this dish ....

Is this dish easy or difficult for you to make?

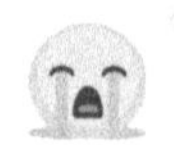 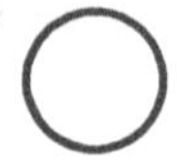 ◯   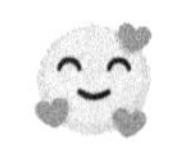 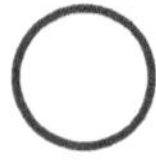 ◯

INGREDIENTS

- 1 cup shredded Swiss cheese
- 1 cup shredded Gruyère cheese
- 2 tbsp all-purpose flour
- 1 clove garlic, minced
- 1 cup dry white wine
- 2 tbsp brandy or kirsch (optional)
- 1/4 tsp ground nutmeg
- 1/4 tsp black pepper

For Dipping:
- Cubed bread
- Apple slices
- Carrot sticks
- Broccoli florets
- Cooked sausage or meatballs

1. In a medium bowl, toss the shredded Swiss and Gruyère cheeses with the flour until well coated.

2. Rub the inside of a fondue pot or medium saucepan with the garlic clove. Discard the garlic.

3. Add the white wine to the fondue pot and heat over medium, stirring occasionally, until steaming but not boiling.

4. Reduce the heat to low and gradually add the cheese mixture, a handful at a time, stirring constantly with a wooden spoon until each addition is fully melted before adding more.

5. Once all the cheese has been incorporated and the fondue is smooth, stir in the brandy (if using) and the nutmeg and black pepper.

6. Keep the fondue warm over a low flame, stirring occasionally, while you prepare the dipping items.

7. Serve the warm cheese fondue immediately, with the assorted dipping items arranged around the fondue pot.

Encourage the teens to spear the dipping items with fondue forks or skewers and swirl them in the melted cheese. This interactive, shareable dish is perfect for a fun group activity.

Did you have fun cooking this dish?

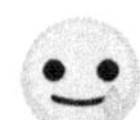 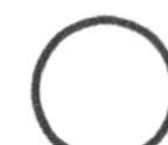 ◯   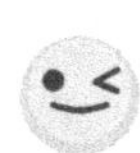 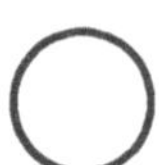 ◯

How would you rate this dish?

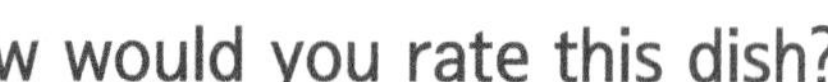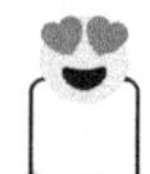 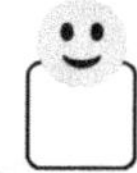 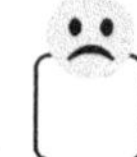  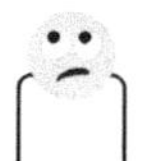 

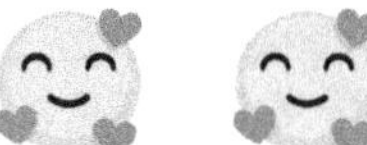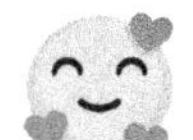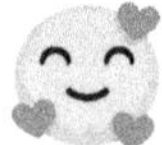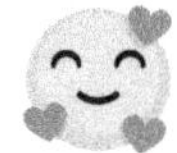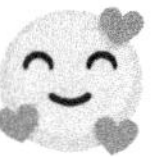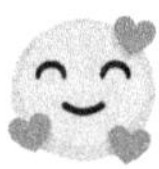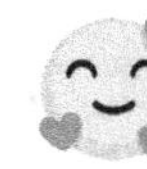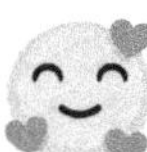

68. Beef sliders

Let's do that and fill in the time here  Prep Time :   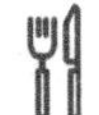 Cook Time :   Servings :

Write 5 friends with whom you want to share this dish
....
....
....
....
....

Is this dish easy or difficult for you to make?

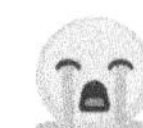 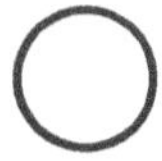 ◯   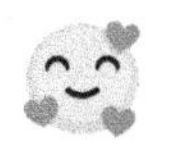 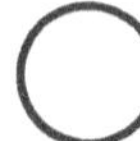 ◯

INGREDIENTS

- 1 lb ground beef
- 1 tsp Worcestershire sauce
- 1 tsp garlic powder
- 1 tsp onion powder
- 1/2 tsp salt
- 1/4 tsp black pepper
- 12 small slider buns or dinner rolls
- Toppings (optional): cheese slices, lettuce, tomato, pickles, ketchup, mustard

1. In a large bowl, gently mix together the ground beef, Worcestershire sauce, garlic powder, onion powder, salt, and pepper until just combined. Be careful not to overmix.

2. Divide the beef mixture into 12 equal portions and shape them into small, flat patties, about 2-3 inches wide.

3. Heat a large skillet or griddle over medium-high heat. Working in batches if needed, cook the slider patties for 2-3 minutes per side, until cooked through.

4. Place the cooked slider patties on the bottom halves of the buns. Top with your desired toppings.

5. Place the top buns on the sliders and serve immediately.

Tip: For extra flavor, you can toast the buns lightly before assembling the sliders.

These mini beef sliders are perfect for young teens. They're easy to hold and eat, and the small size makes them great for sampling different topping combinations. The simple seasoning lets the beef flavor shine through. Offer a variety of toppings so they can customize their sliders.

Did you have fun cooking this dish?

 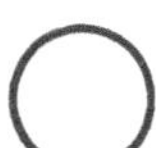 ◯    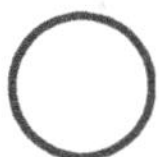 ◯

How would you rate this dish?

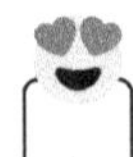 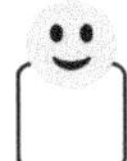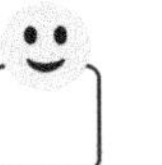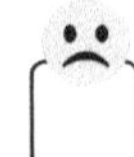 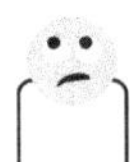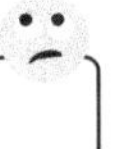 

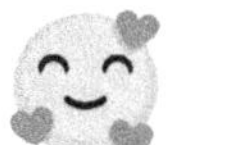 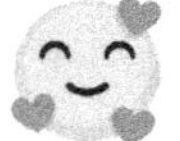 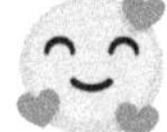 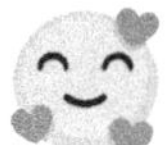 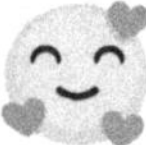 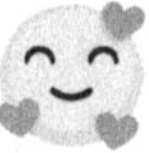  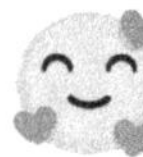  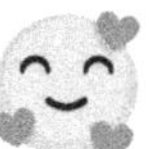

69. Pepperoni calzone

Let's do that and fill in the time here  Prep Time :   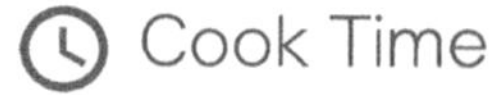 Cook Time :   Servings :

Write 5 friends with whom you want to share this dish
....
....
....
....
....

INGREDIENTS

- 1 lb pizza dough, store-bought or homemade
- 1 cup shredded mozzarella cheese
- 1/2 cup grated Parmesan cheese
- 1 cup diced pepperoni
- 1 cup marinara sauce, for dipping

For the Egg Wash:
- 1 egg, beaten with 1 tbsp water

Is this dish easy or difficult for you to make?

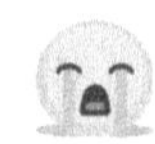 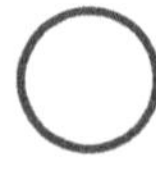 ◯    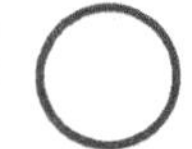 ◯

1. Preheat your oven to 400°F. Line a baking sheet with parchment paper.

2. Divide the pizza dough into 4 equal pieces. On a lightly floured surface, roll each piece into a 6-inch circle.

3. In a small bowl, mix together the mozzarella cheese, Parmesan cheese, and diced pepperoni.

4. Place about 1/4 of the cheese and pepperoni mixture onto the center of each dough circle, leaving a 1-inch border.

5. Fold the dough over the filling to create a half-moon shape. Crimp and seal the edges with a fork.

6. Place the calzones on the prepared baking sheet. Brush the tops with the egg wash.

7. Bake for 18-22 minutes, until the calzones are golden brown.

8. Serve the warm pepperoni calzones with the marinara sauce for dipping.

These pepperoni calzones are perfect for young teens - they're portable, easy to eat, and full of cheesy, pepperoni goodness. The egg wash gives them a nice golden brown crust. Serve them with marinara sauce for dipping.

Did you have fun cooking this dish?

  ◯   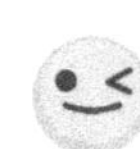 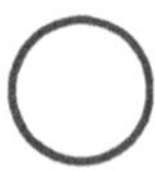 ◯

How would you rate this dish?

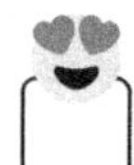 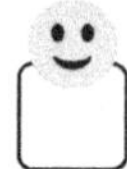  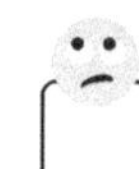 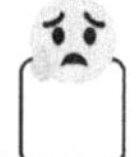

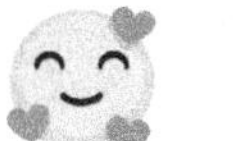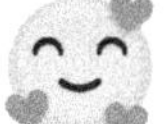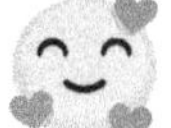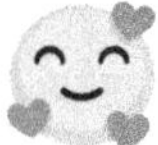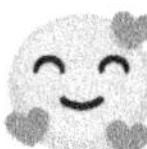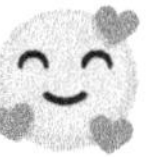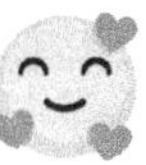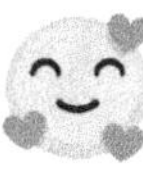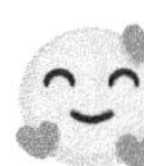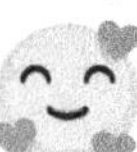

70. Buffalo chicken dip

Let's do that and fill in the time here ✅ Prep Time :   🕐 Cook Time :   🍴 Servings :

Write 5 friends with whom you want to share this dish
....
....
....
....
....

INGREDIENTS

- 2 cups shredded cooked chicken
- 8 oz cream cheese, softened
- 1/2 cup hot sauce (such as Frank's RedHot)
- 1/2 cup ranch dressing
- 1 cup shredded cheddar cheese
- 1/4 cup crumbled blue cheese (optional)
- Tortilla chips, crackers, or celery sticks for serving

Is this dish easy or difficult for you to make?

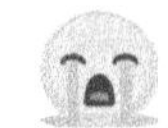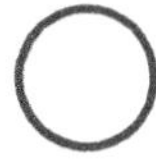 ◯   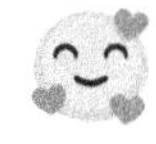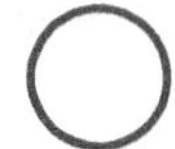 ◯

1. Preheat your oven to 350°F. Grease a 9-inch baking dish.

2. In a large bowl, mix together the shredded chicken, softened cream cheese, hot sauce, and ranch dressing until well combined.

3. Stir in the shredded cheddar cheese and crumbled blue cheese (if using).

4. Transfer the buffalo chicken dip mixture to the prepared baking dish.

5. Bake for 20-25 minutes, until the dip is hot and bubbly.

6. Remove the dip from the oven and let it cool for 5 minutes.

7. Serve the warm buffalo chicken dip immediately with tortilla chips, crackers, or celery sticks for dipping.

This buffalo chicken dip is a crowd-pleasing appetizer that young teens will love. The combination of spicy hot sauce, creamy cheeses, and tender chicken is irresistible. Serve it with plenty of crunchy dippers for maximum enjoyment.

Did you have fun cooking this dish?

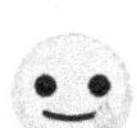 ◯   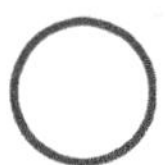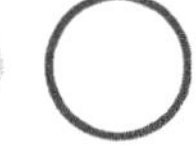 ◯

How would you rate this dish?

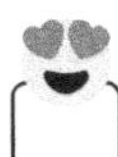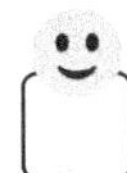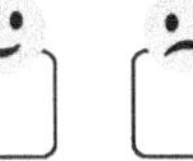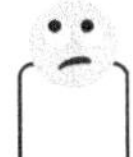

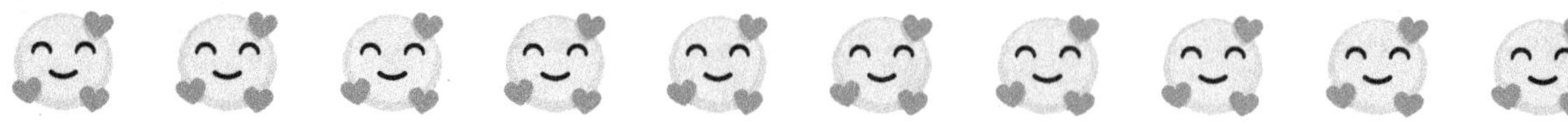

71. Cheesy potato wedges

 Prep Time : 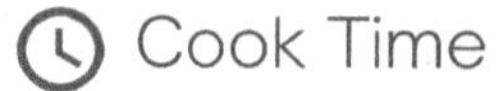 Cook Time : 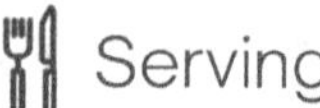 Servings :

Write 5 friends with whom you want to share this dish

Is this dish easy or difficult for you to make?

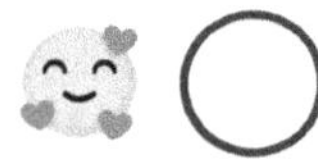 ⃝   ⃝

INGREDIENTS

- 4 medium russet potatoes, washed and cut into 8 wedges each
- 2 tbsp olive oil
- 1 tsp garlic powder
- 1 tsp paprika
- 1/2 tsp salt
- 1/4 tsp black pepper
- 1 cup shredded cheddar cheese
- 2 tbsp chopped fresh parsley (optional)

1. Preheat your oven to 400°F. Line a large baking sheet with parchment paper.

2. In a large bowl, toss the potato wedges with the olive oil, garlic powder, paprika, salt, and pepper until evenly coated.

3. Arrange the seasoned potato wedges in a single layer on the prepared baking sheet.

4. Bake for 25-30 minutes, flipping the wedges halfway through, until they are golden brown and tender.

5. Remove the baked potato wedges from the oven and sprinkle the shredded cheddar cheese evenly over the top.

6. Return the cheesy potato wedges to the oven for 5 more minutes, until the cheese is melted.

7. Garnish the cheesy potato wedges with chopped fresh parsley, if desired.

8. Serve the warm, cheesy potato wedges immediately.

These cheesy potato wedges are a delicious and satisfying snack or side dish that young teens will love. The crispy baked potatoes topped with melty cheddar cheese are irresistible. Adjust the seasonings to your teens' tastes.

Did you have fun cooking this dish?

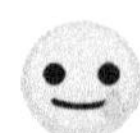 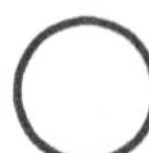 ⃝    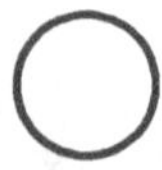 ⃝

How would you rate this dish?

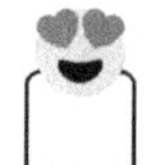 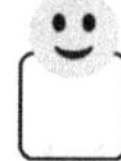 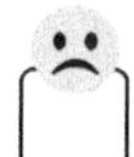 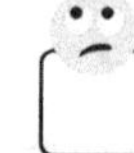 

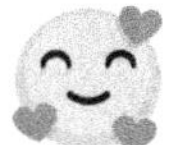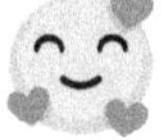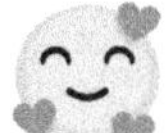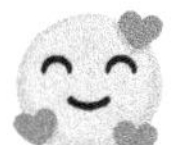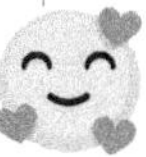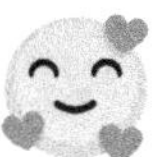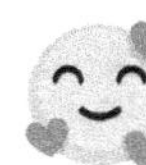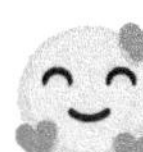

72. Chicken enchiladas

 *Let's do that and fill in the time here* **Prep Time :**   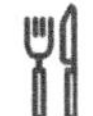 **Cook Time :**   **Servings :**

Write 5 friends with whom you want to share this dish
....
....
....
....
....

Is this dish easy or difficult for you to make?

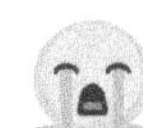 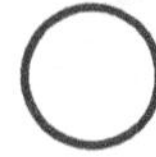 ◯   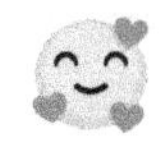 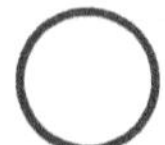 ◯

INGREDIENTS

- 2 cups cooked, shredded chicken
- 1 (15 oz) can black beans, drained and rinsed
- 1 cup shredded cheddar or Monterey Jack cheese
- 1/2 cup sour cream
- 1 (10 oz) can enchilada sauce
- 8 small flour tortillas

Toppings (optional):
- Diced tomatoes
- Sliced green onions
- Chopped cilantro
- Shredded lettuce

1. Preheat your oven to 350°F. Grease a 9x13 inch baking dish.

2. In a large bowl, mix together the shredded chicken, black beans, 1/2 cup of the shredded cheese, and the sour cream.

3. Spread about 1/4 cup of the enchilada sauce in the bottom of the prepared baking dish.

4. Place about 1/3 cup of the chicken mixture onto the center of each tortilla. Roll up the tortilla and place it seam-side down in the baking dish.

5. Pour the remaining enchilada sauce over the top of the rolled enchiladas.

6. Sprinkle the remaining 1/2 cup of shredded cheese over the top.

7. Bake for 20-25 minutes, until the cheese is melted and bubbly.

8. Serve the chicken enchiladas warm, topped with any desired toppings like diced tomatoes, sliced green onions, chopped cilantro, or shredded lettuce.

These chicken enchiladas are a crowd-pleasing meal that young teens will love. The combination of tender chicken, beans, cheese, and enchilada sauce is so satisfying. Plus, they're easy to customize with their favorite toppings.

Did you have fun cooking this dish?

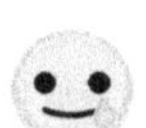 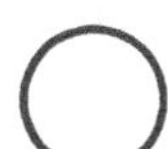 ◯   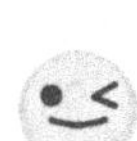  ◯

How would you rate this dish?

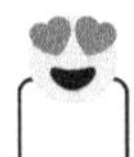 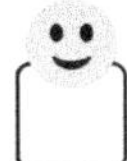 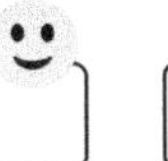 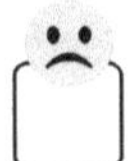 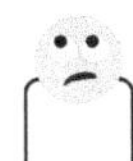 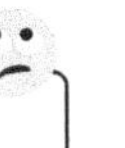 

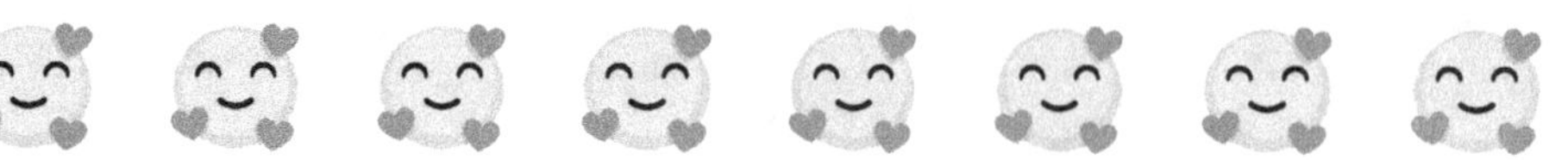

73. Beef empanadas

 Prep Time : 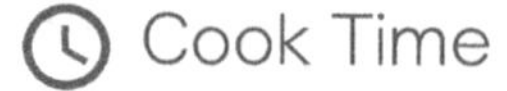 Cook Time :  Servings :

Write 5 friends with whom you want to share this dish

....
....
....
....
....

INGREDIENTS

- 1 lb ground beef
- 1 onion, finely chopped
- 2 cloves garlic, minced
- 1 tsp ground cumin
- 1 tsp dried oregano
- 1/2 tsp smoked paprika
- 1/4 tsp cayenne pepper (optional)
- Salt and pepper to taste
- 1 package refrigerated pie crust or empanada dough
- 1 egg, beaten with 1 tbsp water for egg wash

Is this dish easy or difficult for you to make?

1. In a large skillet over medium heat, cook the ground beef, onion, and garlic until the beef is browned and the onion is softened, about 5-7 minutes. Drain any excess fat.

2. Stir in the cumin, oregano, smoked paprika, and cayenne (if using). Season with salt and pepper to taste. Allow the filling to cool slightly.

3. Preheat your oven to 400°F. Line a baking sheet with parchment paper.

4. On a lightly floured surface, roll out the pie crust or empanada dough to about 1/8-inch thickness. Use a 4-inch round cookie cutter or biscuit cutter to cut out circles.

5. Place about 2-3 tablespoons of the beef filling in the center of each dough circle. Fold the dough over to form a half-moon shape and crimp the edges with a fork to seal.

6. Transfer the empanadas to the prepared baking sheet. Brush the tops with the egg wash.

7. Bake for 18-22 minutes, until the empanadas are golden brown.

8. Serve the warm beef empanadas immediately.

These beef empanadas are a delicious and portable snack that young teens will love. The flaky pastry and savory beef filling make them irresistible. Adjust the spice level to your teens' preferences.

Did you have fun cooking this dish?

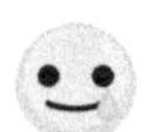   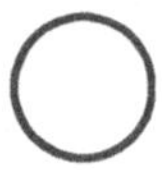

How would you rate this dish?

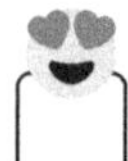 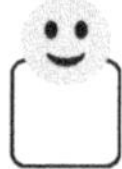  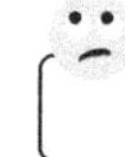 

 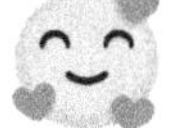 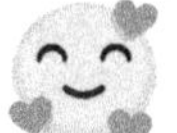 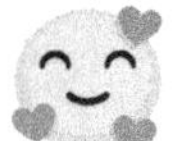 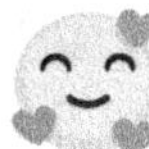 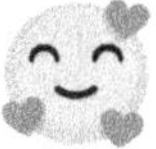 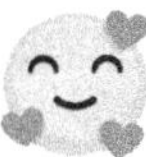 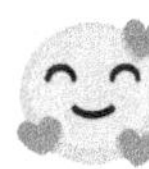  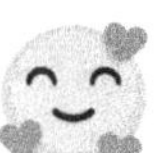

74. Loaded tater tots

Let's do that and fill in the time here  Prep Time :   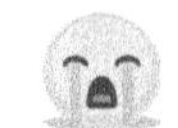 Cook Time :   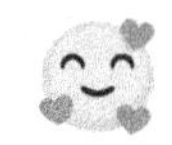 Servings :

Write 5 friends with whom you want to share this dish ....

Is this dish easy or difficult for you to make?

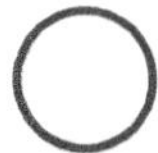 ◯   ◯ 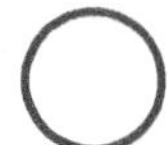

INGREDIENTS

- 1 (32 oz) bag frozen tater tots
- 1 cup shredded cheddar cheese
- 6 slices bacon, cooked and crumbled
- 2 green onions, sliced
- Sour cream, for serving (optional)

1. Preheat your oven to 400°F. Line a large baking sheet with parchment paper.

2. Spread the frozen tater tots in a single layer on the prepared baking sheet.

3. Bake the tater tots for 20-25 minutes, flipping halfway, until golden brown and crispy.

4. Remove the baked tater tots from the oven and top them evenly with the shredded cheddar cheese.

5. Return the cheesy tater tots to the oven for 5 more minutes, until the cheese is melted.

6. Sprinkle the crumbled bacon and sliced green onions over the top of the loaded tater tots.

7. Serve the warm, loaded tater tots immediately, with sour cream on the side for dipping, if desired.

These loaded tater tots are a fun and tasty snack that young teens will love. The crispy tater tots are topped with melty cheddar cheese, crispy bacon, and fresh green onions for a flavor-packed bite. The sour cream adds a cool, creamy contrast.

You can easily customize the toppings to your teens' preferences. Other topping ideas include diced tomatoes, jalapeños, chives, or even chili and cheese.

Did you have fun cooking this dish?

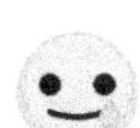 ◯    ◯

How would you rate this dish?

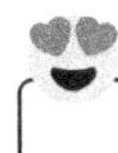 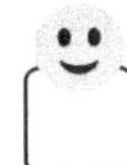 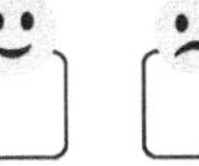  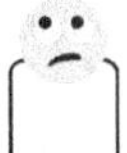 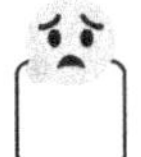

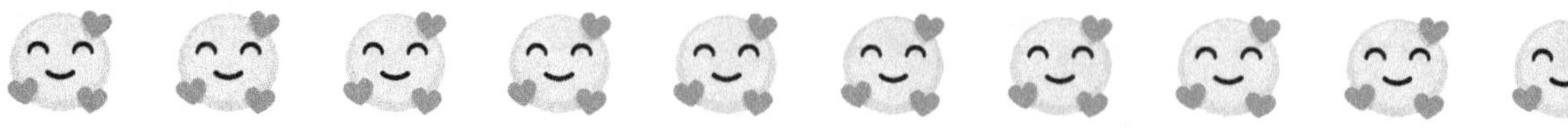

75. Chicken and waffles

 Prep Time :  Cook Time : Servings :

Let's do that and fill in the time here

Write 5 friends with whom you want to share this dish

....

....

....

....

....

Is this dish easy or difficult for you to make?

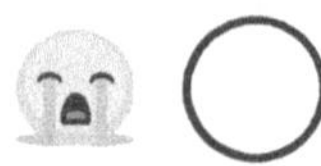 ◯ 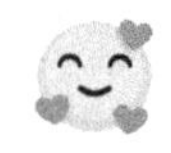 ◯

INGREDIENTS

For the Chicken:
- 1 lb boneless, skinless chicken tenders
- 1 cup buttermilk
- 1 cup all-purpose flour
- 1 tsp paprika
- 1 tsp garlic powder
- 1/2 tsp salt
- 1/4 tsp black pepper
- Vegetable oil for frying

For the Waffles:
- 1 1/2 cups all-purpose flour
- 1 tbsp white sugar
- 2 tsp baking powder
- 1/2 tsp salt
- 1 1/4 cups milk
- 1/3 cup vegetable oil
- 1 egg

1. Place the chicken tenders in a shallow dish and pour the buttermilk over them, turning to coat. Cover and refrigerate for at least 30 minutes (or up to 2 hours).

2. In a shallow bowl, mix together the flour, paprika, garlic powder, salt, and pepper.

3. Remove the chicken from the buttermilk one piece at a time and dredge it in the seasoned flour, pressing to help the coating adhere.

4. In a large skillet or Dutch oven, heat 1-2 inches of vegetable oil to 350°F.

5. Working in batches, carefully add the breaded chicken to the hot oil and fry for 3-4 minutes per side, until golden brown and cooked through.

6. Transfer the fried chicken to a paper towel-lined plate.

7. In a large bowl, whisk together the flour, sugar, baking powder, and salt for the waffles.

8. In a separate bowl, whisk together the milk, vegetable oil, and egg.

9. Pour the wet ingredients into the dry ingredients and stir just until combined (do not overmix).

10. Cook the waffles in a preheated waffle iron according to the manufacturer's instructions.

11. Serve the warm fried chicken tenders on top of the freshly made waffles. Drizzle with maple syrup, if desired.

Did you have fun cooking this dish?

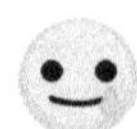 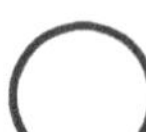 ◯  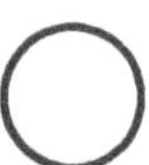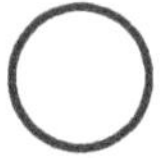 ◯

How would you rate this dish?

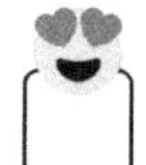 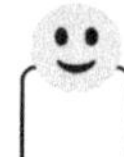 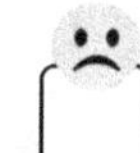 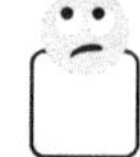 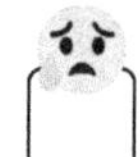

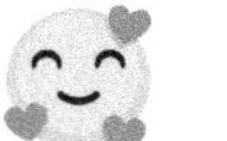 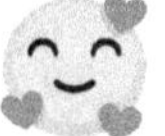 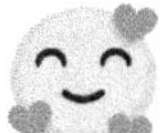 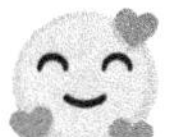 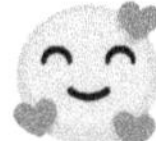 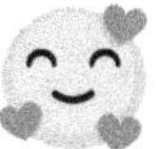 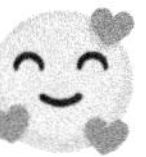 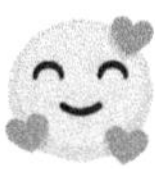  

76. Beef chili

Let's do that and fill in the time here 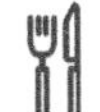 Prep Time :   Cook Time :   Servings :

Write 5 friends with whom you want to share this dish ....

Is this dish easy or difficult for you to make?

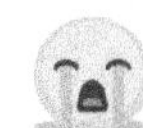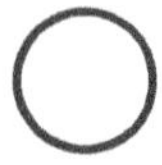 ○   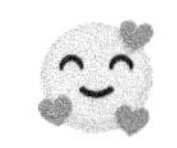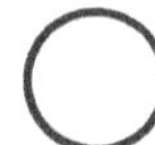 ○

INGREDIENTS

- 1 lb ground beef
- 1 onion, diced
- 3 cloves garlic, minced
- 2 tbsp chili powder
- 1 tsp ground cumin
- 1 tsp dried oregano
- 1/2 tsp smoked paprika
- 1/4 tsp cayenne pepper (optional)
- 1 (15 oz) can diced tomatoes
- 1 (15 oz) can kidney beans, drained and rinsed
- 1 (15 oz) can black beans, drained and rinsed
- 1 cup beef broth
- Salt and pepper to taste

Toppings (optional):
- Shredded cheddar cheese
- Sour cream

1. In a large pot or Dutch oven, cook the ground beef over medium-high heat, breaking it up with a wooden spoon, until browned and cooked through, about 5-7 minutes. Drain any excess fat.

2. Add the diced onion and minced garlic to the pot. Cook for 2-3 minutes, until the onion is translucent.

3. Stir in the chili powder, cumin, oregano, smoked paprika, and cayenne (if using). Cook for 1 minute to toast the spices.

4. Pour in the diced tomatoes, kidney beans, black beans, and beef broth. Stir to combine.

5. Bring the chili to a simmer and let it cook for 20-25 minutes, stirring occasionally, until thickened to your desired consistency.

6. Season the chili with salt and pepper to taste.

7. Serve the beef chili warm, with desired toppings such as shredded cheddar cheese, sour cream, diced onions, and tortilla chips.

This hearty beef chili is sure to be a hit with young teens. The combination of ground beef, beans, and spices creates a flavorful and satisfying dish. Offer a variety of toppings so they can customize their chili.

Did you have fun cooking this dish?

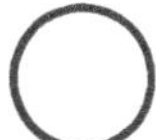 ○   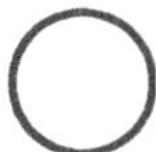 ○

How would you rate this dish?

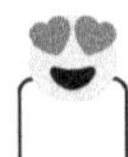 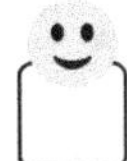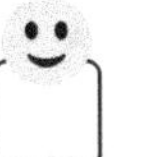 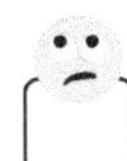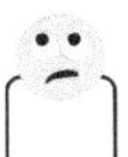 

77. Pizza pockets

 Prep Time : 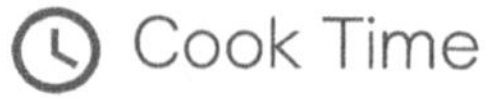  Cook Time : Servings :

Is this dish easy or difficult for you to make?

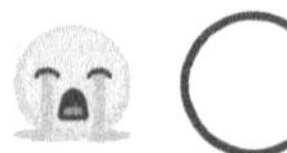 ◯  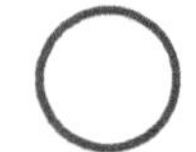 ◯

Write 5 friends with whom you want to share this dish

INGREDIENTS

- 1 lb pizza dough, store-bought or homemade
- 1 cup shredded mozzarella cheese
- 1/2 cup pepperoni slices, chopped
- 1/2 cup diced bell peppers (optional)
- 1/2 cup diced onions (optional)
- 1 cup marinara sauce, for dipping

For the Egg Wash:
- 1 egg, beaten with 1 tbsp water

1. Preheat your oven to 400°F. Line a baking sheet with parchment paper.

2. Divide the pizza dough into 8 equal pieces. On a lightly floured surface, roll each piece into a 5-inch circle.

3. In the center of each dough circle, place about 2 tablespoons of the shredded mozzarella cheese, 1-2 tablespoons of chopped pepperoni, and any other desired toppings like diced bell peppers or onions.

4. Fold the dough over the filling to create a half-moon shape. Crimp and seal the edges with a fork.

5. Place the pizza pockets on the prepared baking sheet. Brush the tops with the egg wash.

6. Bake for 18-22 minutes, until the pizza pockets are golden brown.

7. Serve the warm pizza pockets with the marinara sauce for dipping.

These pizza pockets are a fun and portable snack that young teens will love. The combination of melty cheese, pepperoni, and other toppings inside the crispy dough is irresistible. Encourage them to customize the fillings to their preferences.

Did you have fun cooking this dish?

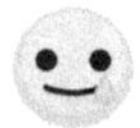 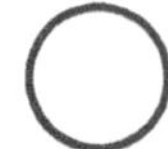 ◯  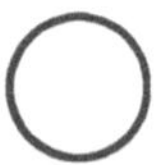 ◯

How would you rate this dish?

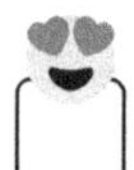    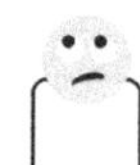 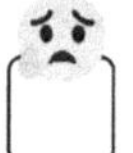

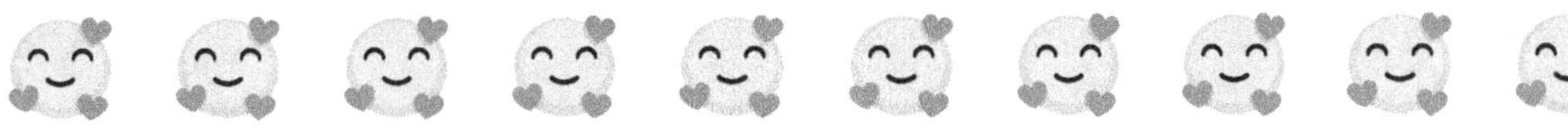

78. Fried chicken sandwich

 Prep Time :   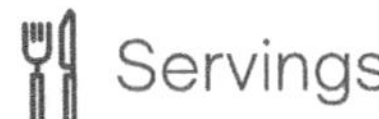 Cook Time :   Servings :

Is this dish easy or difficult for you to make?

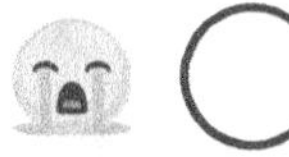 ◯   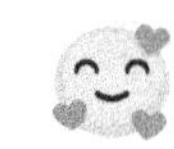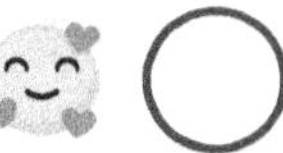 ◯

Write 5 friends with whom you want to share this dish

....

....

....

....

....

INGREDIENTS

- 4 boneless, skinless chicken breasts, pounded thin
- 1 cup buttermilk
- 1 cup all-purpose flour
- 1 tsp paprika
- 1 tsp garlic powder
- 1 tsp salt
- 1/2 tsp black pepper
- Vegetable oil for frying
- 4 brioche or potato hamburger buns, toasted
- Toppings (optional): pickles, lettuce, tomato, mayonnaise, hot sauce

1. Place the chicken breasts in a shallow dish and pour the buttermilk over them, turning to coat. Cover and refrigerate for at least 30 minutes (or up to 2 hours).

2. In a shallow bowl, mix together the flour, paprika, garlic powder, salt, and pepper.

3. Remove the chicken from the buttermilk one piece at a time and dredge it in the seasoned flour, pressing to help the coating adhere.

4. In a large skillet or Dutch oven, heat 1-2 inches of vegetable oil to 350°F.

5. Working in batches, carefully add the breaded chicken to the hot oil and fry for 3-4 minutes per side, until golden brown and cooked through.

6. Transfer the fried chicken to a paper towel-lined plate.

7. Place a fried chicken breast on the bottom half of each toasted bun. Top with your desired toppings.

8. Serve the fried chicken sandwiches immediately.

These crispy, juicy fried chicken sandwiches are sure to be a hit with young teens. The buttermilk marinade and seasoned flour coating make the chicken extra flavorful. Let them customize their sandwiches with their favorite toppings.

Did you have fun cooking this dish?

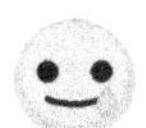 ◯   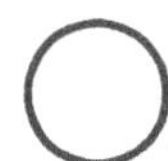 ◯

How would you rate this dish?

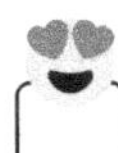 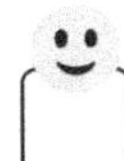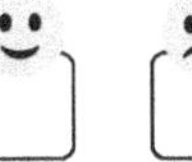  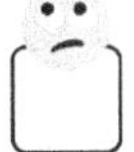 

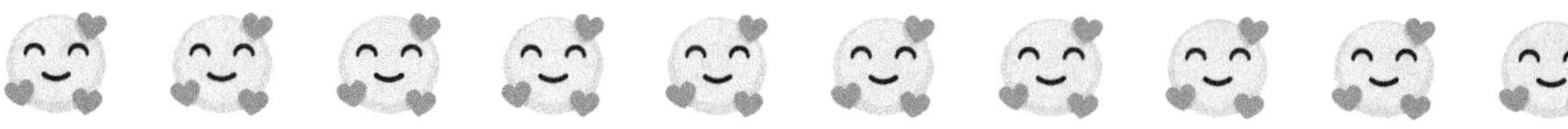

79. Cheese-stuffed meatballs

 *Let's do that and fill in the time here*   Prep Time :

Cook Time :   Servings :

Write 5 friends with whom you want to share this dish

....
....
....
....
....

Is this dish easy or difficult for you to make?

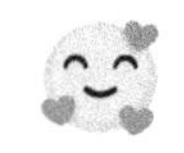 ◯   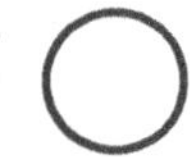 ◯

INGREDIENTS

- 1 lb ground beef
- 1/2 cup breadcrumbs
- 1/4 cup grated Parmesan cheese
- 1 egg
- 2 cloves garlic, minced
- 1 tsp dried oregano
- 1/2 tsp salt
- 1/4 tsp black pepper
- 12 cubes of mozzarella cheese (about 1/2 inch each)
- 1 (24 oz) jar marinara sauce

1. Preheat your oven to 400°F. Line a baking sheet with parchment paper.

2. In a large bowl, combine the ground beef, breadcrumbs, Parmesan cheese, egg, garlic, oregano, salt, and pepper. Mix until just combined, being careful not to overmix.

3. Scoop out about 2 tablespoons of the beef mixture and flatten it into a patty in the palm of your hand. Place one cube of mozzarella cheese in the center, then gently wrap the beef around the cheese to fully enclose it.

4. Place the stuffed meatball on the prepared baking sheet. Repeat with the remaining beef mixture and cheese cubes.

5. Bake the stuffed meatballs for 18-22 minutes, until the beef is cooked through.

6. In a large saucepan, heat the marinara sauce over medium heat.

7. Carefully transfer the baked meatballs to the saucepan with the marinara sauce. Gently toss to coat.

8. Serve the warm cheese-stuffed meatballs immediately, with extra sauce for dipping if desired.

These cheese-stuffed meatballs are a fun and flavorful dish that young teens will love. The melty mozzarella center is a delightful surprise in each bite.

Did you have fun cooking this dish?

  ◯    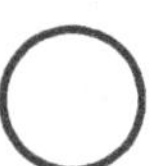 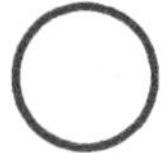 ◯

How would you rate this dish?

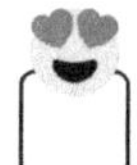 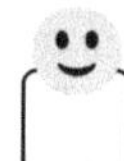  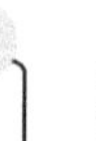 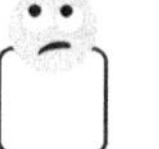 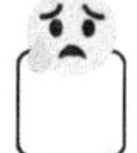

80. BBQ chicken wings

 Prep Time :   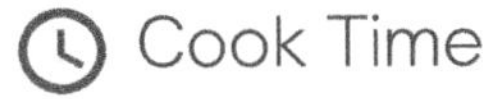 Cook Time :    Servings :

Write 5 friends with whom you want to share this dish

....

....

....

....

....

INGREDIENTS

- 2 lbs chicken wings, drumettes and flats separated
- 1/2 cup barbecue sauce
- 2 tbsp brown sugar
- 1 tsp garlic powder
- 1 tsp onion powder
- 1/2 tsp smoked paprika
- 1/4 tsp cayenne pepper (optional)
- Salt and pepper to taste

Is this dish easy or difficult for you to make?

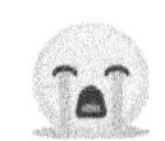 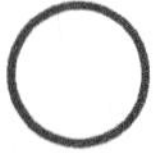 ◯   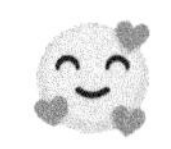 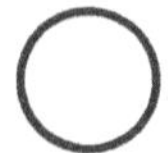 ◯

1. Preheat your oven to 400°F. Line a large baking sheet with parchment paper.

2. In a large bowl, toss the chicken wing pieces with the barbecue sauce, brown sugar, garlic powder, onion powder, smoked paprika, and cayenne pepper (if using). Season with salt and pepper.

3. Arrange the coated chicken wings in a single layer on the prepared baking sheet.

4. Bake for 30-35 minutes, flipping the wings halfway through, until they are cooked through and crispy.

5. For extra caramelization, you can broil the wings for 2-3 minutes at the end, watching carefully to prevent burning.

6. Serve the hot BBQ chicken wings immediately, with extra barbecue sauce for dipping if desired.

These BBQ chicken wings are a crowd-pleasing snack that young teens will love. The sweet and savory sauce, combined with the crispy baked skin, makes them irresistible. Adjust the spice level to your teens' preferences.

Did you have fun cooking this dish?

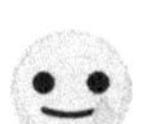  ◯    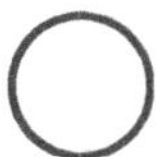 ◯

How would you rate this dish?

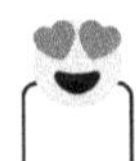 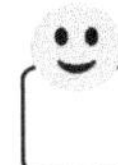 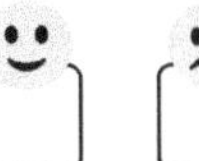  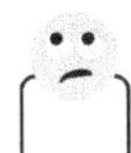 

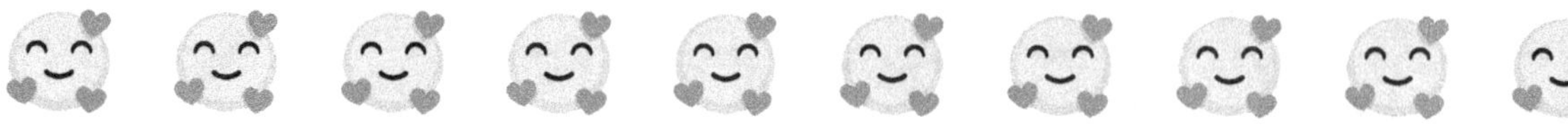

81. Loaded fries

 Prep Time : 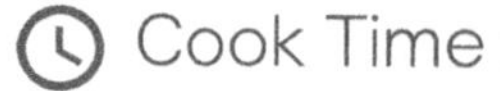 Cook Time : 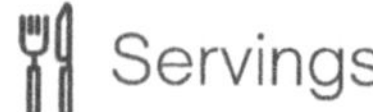 Servings :

Write 5 friends with whom you want to share this dish

....
....
....
....
....

INGREDIENTS

- 2 lbs russet potatoes, cut into 1/4-inch thick fries
- 2 tbsp vegetable oil
- 1 tsp salt
- 1/2 tsp black pepper
- 1 cup shredded cheddar cheese
- 6 slices bacon, cooked and crumbled
- 2 green onions, sliced
- Sour cream, for serving (optional)

Did you have fun cooking this dish?

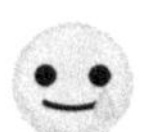 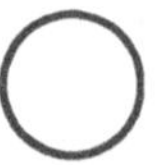

How would you rate this dish?

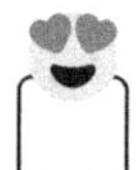 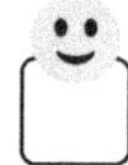 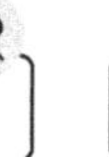 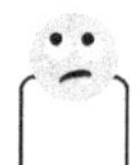 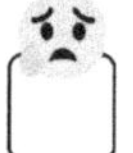

Is this dish easy or difficult for you to make?

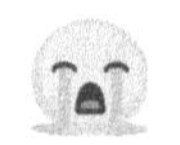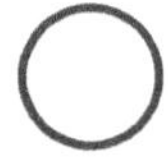 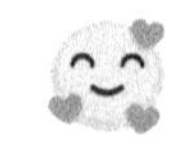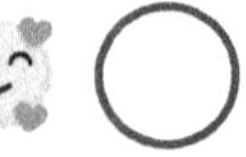

1. Preheat your oven to 400°F. Line a large baking sheet with parchment paper.

2. Place the cut potato fries in a large bowl. Drizzle with the vegetable oil and season with salt and pepper. Toss to coat.

3. Spread the seasoned fries in a single layer on the prepared baking sheet.

4. Bake for 25-30 minutes, flipping the fries halfway, until they are golden brown and crispy.

5. Remove the baked fries from the oven and top them evenly with the shredded cheddar cheese.

6. Return the cheesy fries to the oven for 5 more minutes, until the cheese is melted.

7. Sprinkle the crumbled bacon and sliced green onions over the top of the loaded fries.

8. Serve the warm, loaded fries immediately, with sour cream on the side for dipping, if desired.

These loaded fries are a delicious and satisfying snack that young teens will love. The crispy baked fries are topped with melty cheddar cheese, crispy bacon, and fresh green onions for a flavor-packed treat.

You can easily customize the toppings to your teens' preferences. Other topping ideas include diced tomatoes, jalapeños, chives, or even chili and cheese.

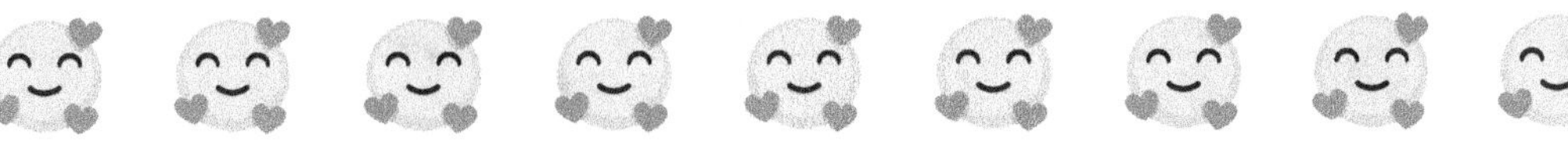

82. Beef and cheese quesadilla

 Prep Time :   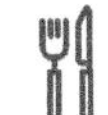 Cook Time :   Servings :

Write 5 friends with whom you want to share this dish

....
....
....
....
....

Is this dish easy or difficult for you to make?

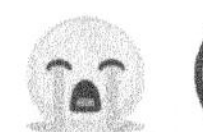 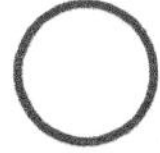 ◯    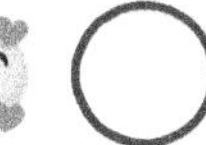 ◯

INGREDIENTS

- 1 lb ground beef
- 1 packet taco seasoning
- 1/2 cup water
- 8 large flour tortillas
- 2 cups shredded cheddar or Monterey Jack cheese
- Salsa, sour cream, and guacamole for serving (optional)

1. In a large skillet, cook the ground beef over medium-high heat, breaking it up with a wooden spoon, until browned and cooked through, about 5-7 minutes. Drain any excess fat.

2. Stir in the taco seasoning and 1/2 cup of water. Simmer for 5 minutes, until the sauce has thickened.

3. Lay 4 of the flour tortillas out on a clean work surface. Divide the seasoned ground beef evenly among the tortillas, spreading it out to cover the surface.

4. Sprinkle the shredded cheese evenly over the beef.

5. Top each quesadilla with the remaining 4 tortillas.

6. Heat a large skillet or griddle over medium heat. Working in batches if needed, cook the quesadillas for 2-3 minutes per side, until the tortillas are golden brown and the cheese is melted.

7. Cut the quesadillas into wedges and serve them warm, with salsa, sour cream, and guacamole on the side for dipping, if desired.

These beef and cheese quesadillas are a crowd-pleasing meal that young teens will love. The combination of seasoned ground beef, melty cheese, and crispy tortillas is always a hit. Encourage them to customize their quesadillas with their favorite toppings.

Did you have fun cooking this dish?

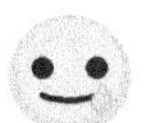  ◯    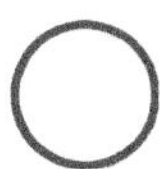 ◯

How would you rate this dish?

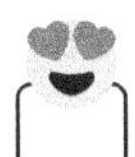 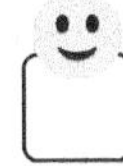 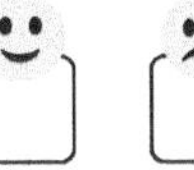 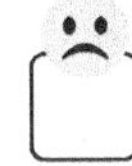 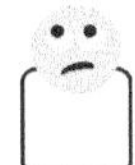 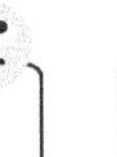 

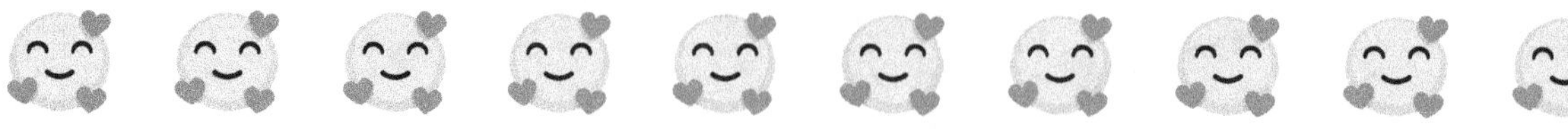

83. Chicken parmesan sliders

 Prep Time : 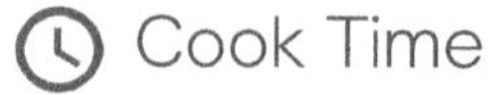 Cook Time : 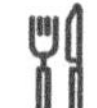 Servings :

Write 5 friends with whom you want to share this dish
....
....
....
....
....

Is this dish easy or difficult for you to make?

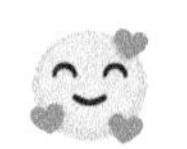 ◯ 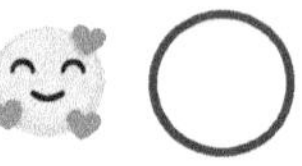 ◯

INGREDIENTS

- 1 lb boneless, skinless chicken breasts
- 1 cup all-purpose flour
- 2 eggs, beaten
- 1 cup panko breadcrumbs
- 1 tsp garlic powder
- 1 tsp Italian seasoning
- 1/2 tsp salt
- 1/4 tsp black pepper
- 1 cup marinara sauce
- 1 cup shredded mozzarella cheese
- 12 small slider buns or dinner rolls, split in half

1. Preheat your oven to 400°F. Line a baking sheet with parchment paper.

2. Pound the chicken breasts between two sheets of plastic wrap or wax paper until they are about 1/2-inch thick. Cut each chicken breast into 3-4 smaller pieces.

3. Set up a breading station with three shallow dishes: one with the flour, one with the beaten eggs, and one with the panko breadcrumbs mixed with the garlic powder, Italian seasoning, salt, and pepper.

4. Dredge the chicken pieces in the flour, then dip them in the egg, and finally coat them in the seasoned panko.

5. Place the breaded chicken pieces on the prepared baking sheet. Bake for 15-18 minutes, flipping halfway, until the chicken is cooked through and crispy.

6. Top each chicken piece with a spoonful of marinara sauce and a sprinkle of mozzarella cheese.

7. Return the chicken to the oven for 5 more minutes, until the cheese is melted.

8. Place the chicken parmesan pieces on the bottom halves of the slider buns. Top with the remaining bun halves.

Serve the warm chicken parmesan sliders immediately.

Did you have fun cooking this dish?

 ◯ 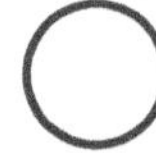  ◯ 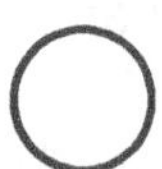

How would you rate this dish?

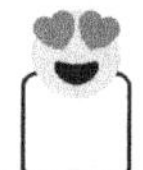 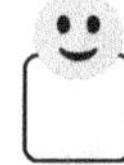  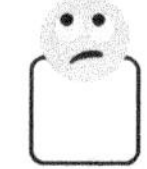 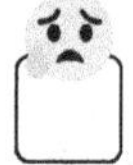

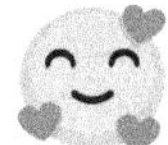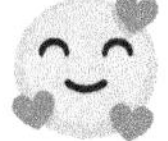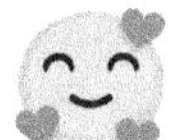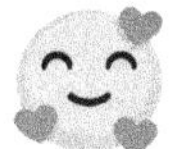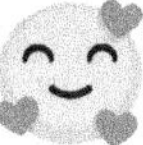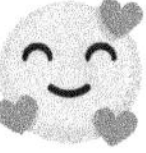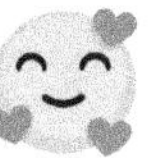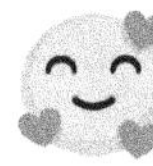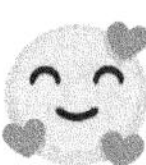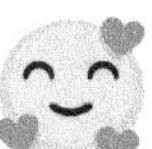

84. Cheesy garlic pull-apart bread

Let's do that and fill in the time here

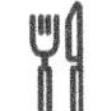 Prep Time :

Cook Time :

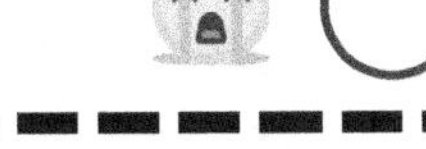 Servings :

Write 5 friends with whom you want to share this dish

....

....

....

....

....

INGREDIENTS

- 1 loaf of unsliced French or Italian bread
- 1/2 cup (1 stick) unsalted butter, melted
- 3 cloves garlic, minced
- 1 tsp dried parsley
- 1/2 tsp salt
- 1/4 tsp black pepper
- 1 1/2 cups shredded mozzarella cheese
- 1/2 cup grated Parmesan cheese

Is this dish easy or difficult for you to make?

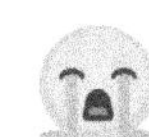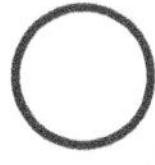 ◯   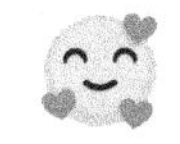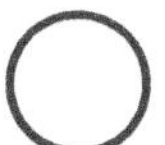 ◯

1. Preheat your oven to 350°F. Grease a 9x13 inch baking dish.

2. Use a serrated knife to cut the bread into 1-inch cubes, making sure not to cut all the way through the bottom crust.

3. In a small bowl, whisk together the melted butter, minced garlic, dried parsley, salt, and black pepper.

4. Drizzle the garlic butter mixture evenly over the cubed bread, making sure to get it in between the cubes.

5. Sprinkle the shredded mozzarella and grated Parmesan cheeses evenly over the top of the bread.

6. Bake for 20-25 minutes, until the cheese is melted and bubbly.

7. Serve the warm cheesy garlic pull-apart bread immediately, allowing guests to pull off the individual cubes.

This cheesy garlic pull-apart bread is a fun and shareable snack that young teens will love. The gooey, melted cheese and garlic-infused bread cubes are irresistible. Encourage them to pull off the individual pieces and enjoy!

Did you have fun cooking this dish?

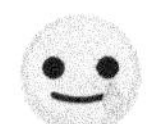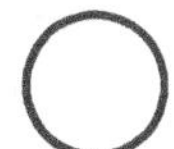 ◯   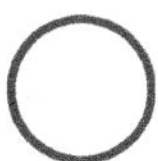 ◯

How would you rate this dish?

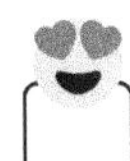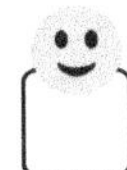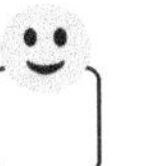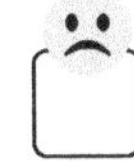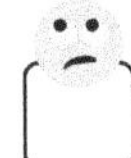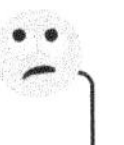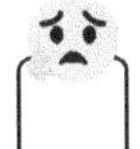

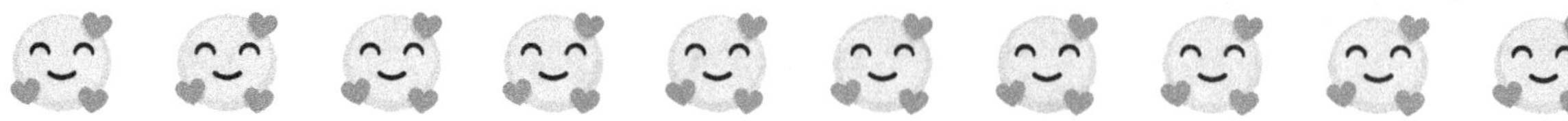

85. Beef and cheddar melt

 Prep Time : 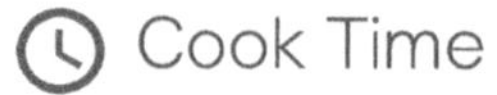 Cook Time :  Servings :

Let's do that and fill in the time here

Write 5 friends with whom you want to share this dish
....
....
....
....
....

INGREDIENTS

- 1 lb ground beef
- 1 onion, diced
- 2 cloves garlic, minced
- 1 tsp Worcestershire sauce
- 1 tsp dried oregano
- 1/2 tsp salt
- 1/4 tsp black pepper
- 8 slices sourdough or brioche bread
- 8 slices cheddar cheese
- 2 tbsp butter, softened

Is this dish easy or difficult for you to make?

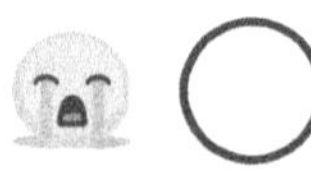 ◯   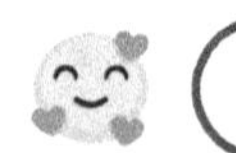 ◯

1. In a large skillet over medium heat, cook the ground beef, onion, and garlic until the beef is browned and the onion is softened, about 5-7 minutes. Drain any excess fat.

2. Stir in the Worcestershire sauce, oregano, salt, and pepper. Remove from heat.

3. Preheat your oven to 400°F. Line a baking sheet with parchment paper.

4. Lay the slices of bread out on a clean work surface. Spread the softened butter evenly on one side of each slice.

5. Place 4 of the bread slices, butter-side down, on the prepared baking sheet. Top each slice with a portion of the seasoned ground beef mixture, followed by a slice of cheddar cheese.

6. Top the sandwiches with the remaining 4 slices of bread, butter-side up.

7. Bake for 10-12 minutes, flipping the sandwiches halfway, until the bread is golden brown and the cheese is melted.

8. Serve the warm beef and cheddar melts immediately.

These beef and cheddar melts are a delicious and satisfying sandwich that young teens will love. The savory beef and melty cheddar cheese are a classic combination. The buttery, toasted bread adds the perfect crunch.

Did you have fun cooking this dish?

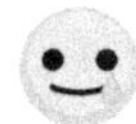 ◯    ◯

How would you rate this dish?

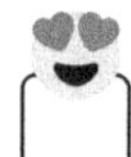   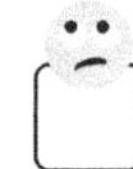 

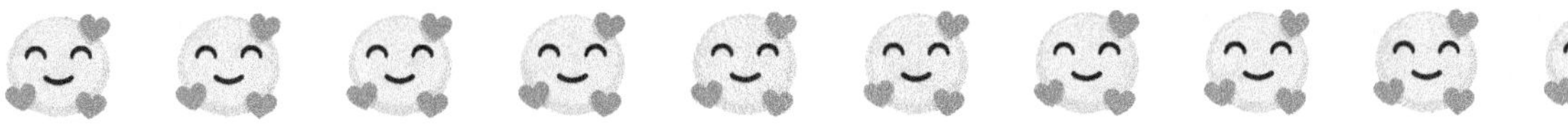

86. Buffalo chicken wrap

Let's do that and fill in the time here  Prep Time :   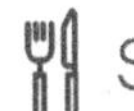 Cook Time :   Servings :

Write 5 friends with whom you want to share this dish

....

....

....

....

....

INGREDIENTS

- 4 boneless, skinless chicken breasts
- 1/2 cup buffalo sauce (such as Frank's RedHot)
- 1/4 cup ranch or blue cheese dressing
- 4 large tortilla or wrap shells
- 1 cup shredded lettuce
- 1/2 cup diced tomatoes
- 1/4 cup crumbled blue cheese (optional)

Is this dish easy or difficult for you to make?

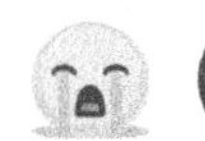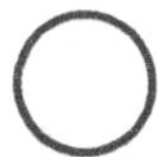 ◯   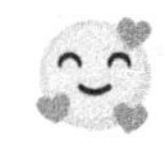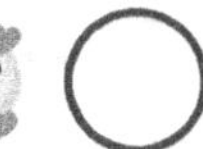 ◯

1. Preheat oven to 400°F. Place the chicken breasts on a baking sheet and bake for 20-25 minutes, until cooked through. Allow to cool slightly, then shred the chicken using two forks.

2. In a bowl, mix the shredded chicken with the buffalo sauce until well coated.

3. Spread 1-2 tablespoons of the ranch or blue cheese dressing down the center of each tortilla or wrap shell.

4. Top with the buffalo chicken mixture, shredded lettuce, diced tomatoes, and crumbled blue cheese (if using).

5. Fold the bottom of the wrap up over the filling, then fold in the sides and continue rolling up tightly.

6. Serve immediately or wrap in foil or parchment paper to enjoy later.

Did you have fun cooking this dish?

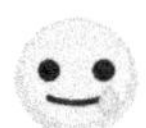 ◯   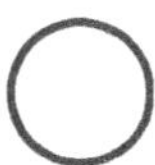 ◯

How would you rate this dish?

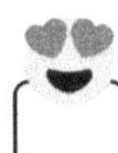   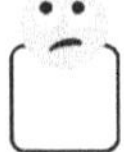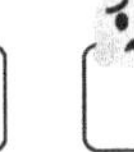

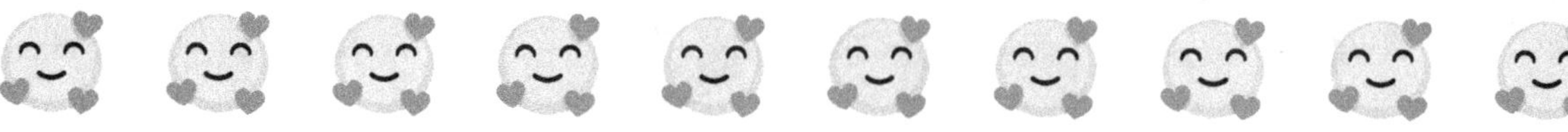

87. Loaded potato soup

 Prep Time : 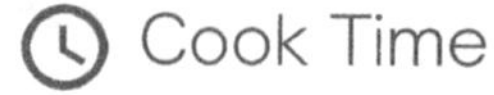 Cook Time : 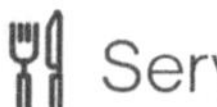 Servings :

Write 5 friends with whom you want to share this dish
....
....
....
....
....

Is this dish easy or difficult for you to make?

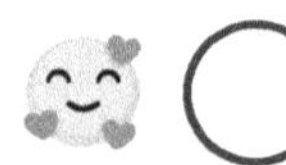 ◯   😊 ◯

INGREDIENTS

- 3 lbs russet potatoes, peeled and diced
- 1 onion, diced
- 3 cloves garlic, minced
- 4 cups chicken or vegetable broth
- 1 cup milk
- 1/2 cup heavy cream
- 1 tsp salt
- 1/2 tsp black pepper
- 1 cup shredded cheddar cheese
- 6 slices bacon, cooked and crumbled
- 2 green onions, sliced

1. In a large pot or Dutch oven, combine the diced potatoes, onion, and garlic. Pour in the broth and bring to a boil over high heat.

2. Reduce the heat to medium-low and simmer the soup for 15-20 minutes, until the potatoes are very tender.

3. Use an immersion blender or regular blender to puree about half of the soup, leaving some potato chunks.

4. Stir in the milk and heavy cream. Season with salt and pepper.

5. Bring the soup back to a simmer and cook for 5 more minutes, until heated through.

6. Ladle the loaded potato soup into bowls and top each serving with shredded cheddar cheese, crumbled bacon, and sliced green onions.

7. Serve the warm, loaded potato soup immediately.

This hearty and comforting loaded potato soup is sure to be a hit with young teens. The creamy, potato-based broth is loaded with all the classic baked potato toppings they love. Adjust the thickness and toppings to their preferences.

Did you have fun cooking this dish?

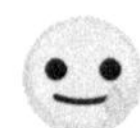 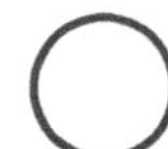 ◯    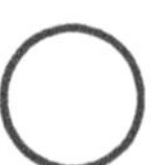 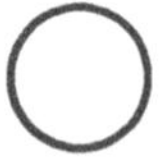 ◯

How would you rate this dish?

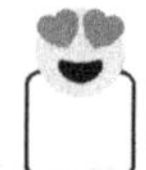 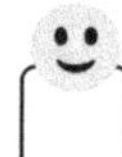  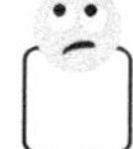 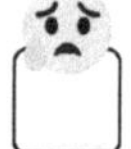

88. Chicken fajita quesadilla

 Prep Time :   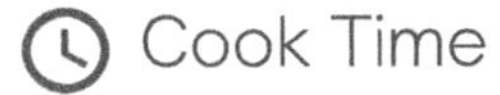 Cook Time :    Servings :

Write 5 friends with whom you want to share this dish

....
....
....
....
....

Is this dish easy or difficult for you to make?

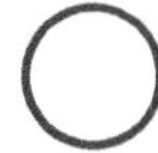 ◯   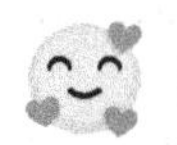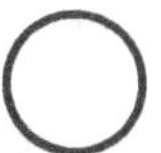 ◯

INGREDIENTS

- 1 lb boneless, skinless chicken breasts, sliced into strips
- 1 tablespoon olive oil
- 1 teaspoon chili powder
- 1 teaspoon cumin
- 1/2 teaspoon garlic powder
- Salt and pepper to taste
- 1 red bell pepper, sliced
- 1 green bell pepper, sliced
- 1 onion, sliced
- 8 medium-sized flour tortillas
- 2 cups shredded Mexican cheese blend

1. In a large skillet, heat the olive oil over medium-high heat. Add the chicken strips and season with the chili powder, cumin, garlic powder, salt, and pepper. Cook for 5-7 minutes, until the chicken is cooked through. Remove from the skillet and set aside.

2. In the same skillet, add the sliced bell peppers and onions. Sauté for 5-7 minutes, until the vegetables are tender and slightly charred.

3. Place one tortilla in the skillet and top with a layer of the cooked chicken, sautéed vegetables, and a handful of shredded cheese. Top with another tortilla.

4. Cook the quesadilla for 2-3 minutes per side, until the tortilla is golden brown and the cheese is melted.

5. Repeat with the remaining tortillas, chicken, vegetables, and cheese to make 4 quesadillas total.

6. Cut each quesadilla into wedges and serve with your favorite toppings like sour cream, salsa, or guacamole.

This recipe is easy to make, full of flavor, and perfect for young teens who love Mexican-inspired dishes. Enjoy!

Did you have fun cooking this dish?

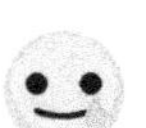 ◯    ◯    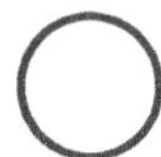

How would you rate this dish?

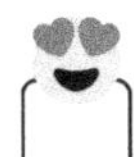 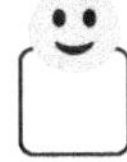 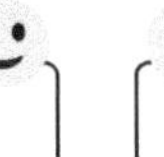  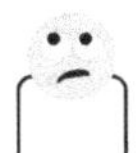  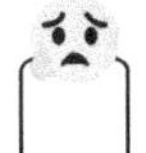

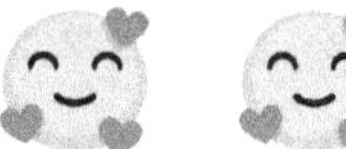 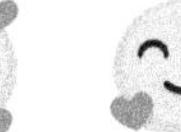 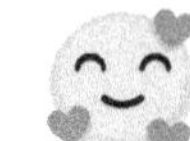 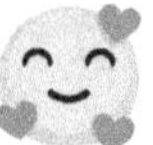 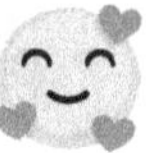 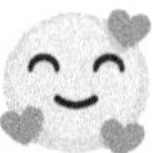 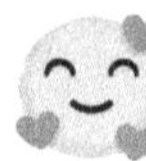 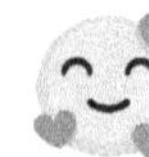 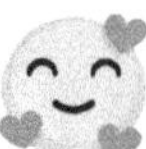

89. Beef taquitos

Let's do that and fill in the time here 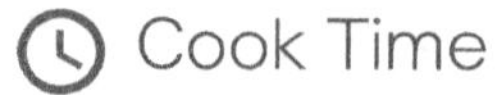 Prep Time :   Cook Time :   Servings :

Write 5 friends with whom you want to share this dish

....

....

....

....

....

INGREDIENTS

- 1 lb ground beef
- 1 packet taco seasoning
- 1/2 cup water
- 12 small corn tortillas
- 1 cup shredded cheddar or Mexican blend cheese
- Vegetable oil for frying
- Toppings (optional): salsa, sour cream, guacamole, etc.

Is this dish easy or difficult for you to make?

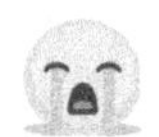 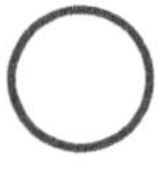 ◯    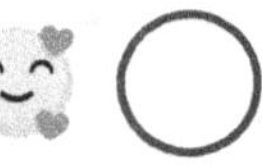 ◯

1. In a skillet over medium heat, cook the ground beef until browned and crumbled, 5-7 minutes. Drain any excess fat.

2. Add the taco seasoning and water to the skillet. Stir and simmer for 2-3 minutes until the sauce thickens.

3. Lay the corn tortillas out on a clean surface. Spoon about 2-3 tablespoons of the beef mixture onto the center of each tortilla. Top with a sprinkle of shredded cheese.

4. Carefully roll up each tortilla tightly around the filling to form a taquito.

5. In a large skillet or Dutch oven, heat about 1/2 inch of vegetable oil over medium-high heat.

6. Working in batches, fry the taquitos for 1-2 minutes per side until golden brown and crispy.

7. Transfer the fried taquitos to a paper towel-lined plate to drain any excess oil.

8. Serve the taquitos warm with your favorite toppings like salsa, sour cream, or guacamole.

These beef taquitos are easy to make, portable, and perfect for young teens to enjoy as a snack or appetizer. The crispy tortilla shell and flavorful beef filling is sure to be a hit!

Did you have fun cooking this dish?

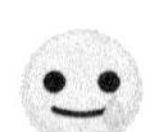 ◯   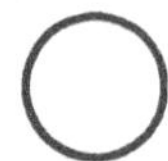 ◯

How would you rate this dish?

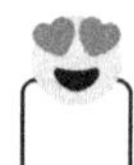 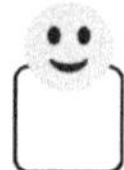 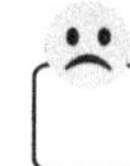 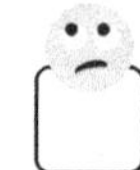 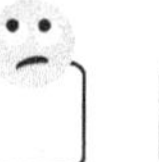 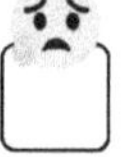

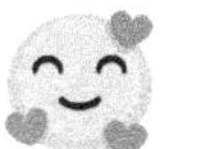 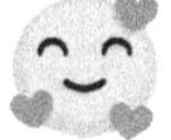 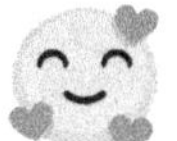 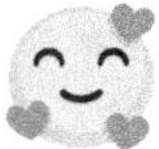 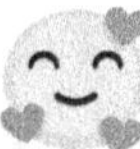 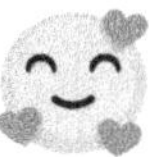 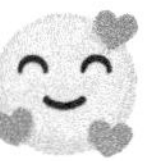 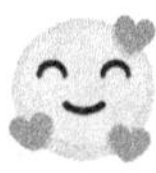 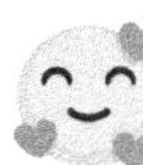 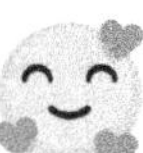

90. Cheese and bacon potato skins

Let's do that and fill in the time here  Prep Time :   Cook Time :   Servings :

Write 5 friends with whom you want to share this dish
....
....
....
....

Is this dish easy or difficult for you to make?

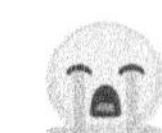 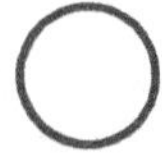 ◯   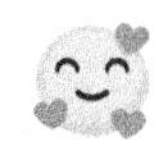 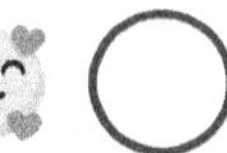 ◯

INGREDIENTS

- 4 medium russet potatoes
- 2 tbsp olive oil
- 1/2 tsp salt
- 1/4 tsp black pepper
- 1 cup shredded cheddar cheese
- 6 slices bacon, cooked and crumbled
- 2 green onions, sliced
- Sour cream for serving (optional)

1. Preheat your oven to 400°F. Wash the potatoes and prick them several times with a fork.

2. Bake the potatoes directly on the oven rack for 50-60 minutes, until they are tender when squeezed. Allow to cool slightly.

3. Cut the potatoes in half lengthwise. Scoop out the insides, leaving about 1/4 inch of potato flesh attached to the skin.

4. Brush the potato skins with the olive oil and season with salt and pepper.

5. Place the potato skins back on the baking sheet, skin-side up. Bake for 10 minutes.

6. Flip the potato skins over and bake for another 10 minutes, until crispy.

7. Remove the potato skins from the oven and top each one with some shredded cheddar cheese and crumbled bacon.

8. Return the loaded potato skins to the oven for 5 more minutes, until the cheese is melted.

9. Garnish the potato skins with the sliced green onions.

10. Serve the warm cheese and bacon potato skins with sour cream on the side for dipping, if desired.

These loaded potato skins are a fun and tasty snack that young teens will love. The crispy potato shells, melty cheese, and crispy bacon make them irresistible.

Did you have fun cooking this dish?

  ◯   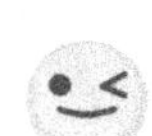 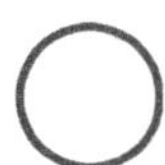 ◯

How would you rate this dish?

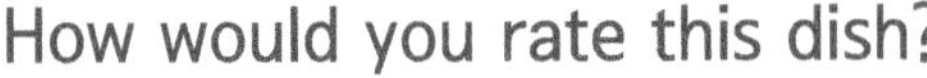
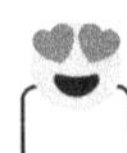 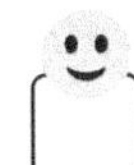   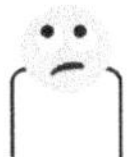 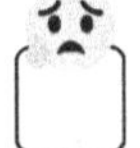

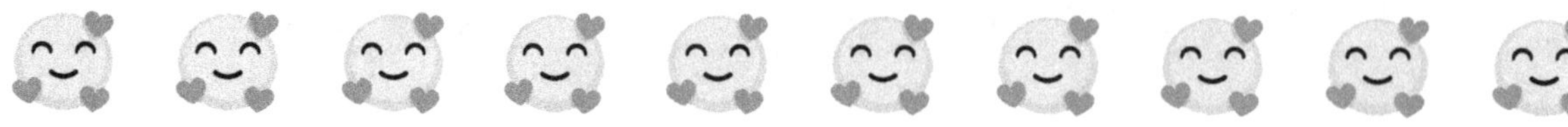

91. BBQ chicken flatbread

 Prep Time : 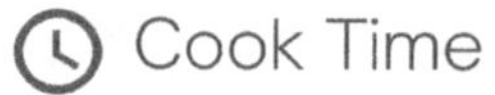 Cook Time : 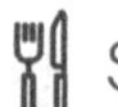 Servings :

Is this dish easy or difficult for you to make?

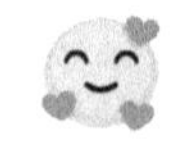 ◯ 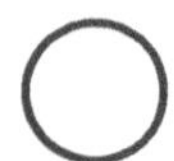 ◯

Write 5 friends with whom you want to share this dish

INGREDIENTS

- 1 lb boneless, skinless chicken breasts
- 1 cup barbecue sauce, divided
- 1 pre-baked flatbread or naan
- 1 cup shredded mozzarella cheese
- 1/2 cup diced red onion
- 2 tablespoons chopped fresh cilantro (optional)

1. Preheat your oven to 400°F.

2. Place the chicken breasts in a baking dish and brush them with 1/4 cup of the barbecue sauce. Bake for 20-25 minutes, until the chicken is cooked through. Allow to cool slightly, then shred the chicken using two forks.

3. In a bowl, mix the shredded chicken with the remaining 3/4 cup of barbecue sauce.

4. Place the flatbread or naan on a baking sheet. Spread the BBQ chicken mixture evenly over the surface, leaving a small border around the edges.

5. Sprinkle the shredded mozzarella cheese over the top of the chicken.

6. Bake the flatbread in the preheated oven for 10-12 minutes, or until the cheese is melted and bubbly.

7. Remove the flatbread from the oven and top with the diced red onion and chopped cilantro (if using).

8. Slice the flatbread into wedges and serve immediately.

This BBQ Chicken Flatbread is a fun and easy-to-eat meal that young teens are sure to love. The combination of the sweet and tangy barbecue sauce, tender chicken, and melty cheese is irresistible. Enjoy!

Did you have fun cooking this dish?

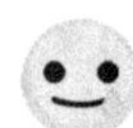 ◯  ◯

How would you rate this dish?

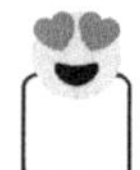 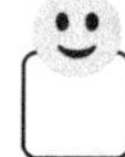 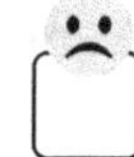  

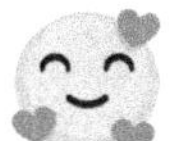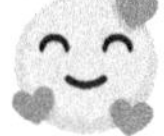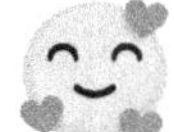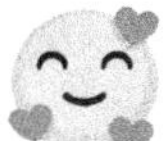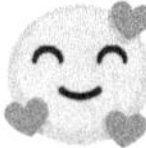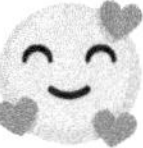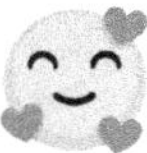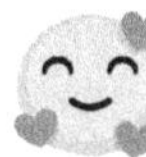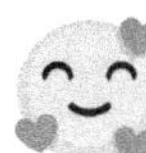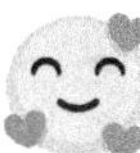

92. Beef and bean chimichanga

Let's do that and fill in the time here

Prep Time :   Cook Time :   Servings :

Write 5 friends with whom you want to share this dish

....
....
....
....
....

INGREDIENTS

- 1 lb ground beef
- 1 packet taco seasoning
- 1 (15 oz) can black beans, drained and rinsed
- 1 cup shredded cheddar cheese
- 8 large flour tortillas
- Vegetable oil for frying
- Toppings (optional): sour cream, salsa, guacamole, etc.

Is this dish easy or difficult for you to make?

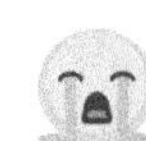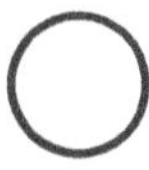 ◯   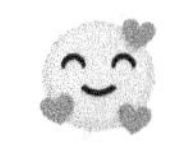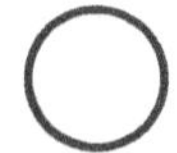 ◯

1. In a large skillet, cook the ground beef over medium heat until browned and crumbled, about 5-7 minutes. Drain any excess fat.

2. Add the taco seasoning and 1/2 cup of water to the skillet. Stir and simmer for 2-3 minutes until the sauce thickens.

3. Remove the skillet from heat and stir in the black beans and 1/2 cup of the shredded cheese.

4. Lay the flour tortillas out on a clean surface. Spoon about 1/3 cup of the beef and bean mixture onto the center of each tortilla.

5. Fold the bottom of the tortilla up over the filling, then fold in the sides and continue rolling up tightly to form a burrito shape.

6. In a large skillet or Dutch oven, heat about 1 inch of vegetable oil over medium-high heat.

7. Working in batches, carefully add the chimichangas to the hot oil and fry for 2-3 minutes per side until golden brown and crispy.

8. Transfer the fried chimichangas to a paper towel-lined plate to drain any excess oil.

9. Serve the chimichangas warm, topped with the remaining shredded cheese and any other desired toppings.

These beef and bean chimichangas are a fun and flavorful Mexican-inspired dish that young teens are sure to love. The crispy fried exterior and savory filling make them irresistible!

Did you have fun cooking this dish?

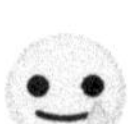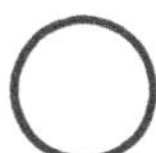 ◯   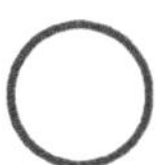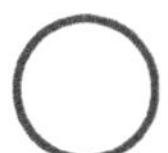 ◯

How would you rate this dish?

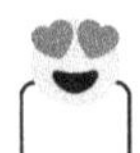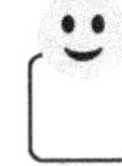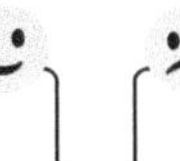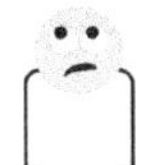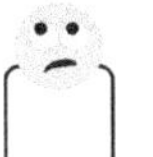

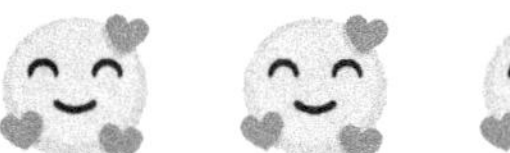

93. Chicken and cheese taquitos

Let's do that and fill in the time here    Prep Time :   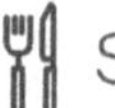 Cook Time :   Servings :

Write 5 friends with whom you want to share this dish ....

Is this dish easy or difficult for you to make?

 ◯    ◯

INGREDIENTS

- 2 cups cooked, shredded chicken
- 1 cup shredded cheddar or Mexican blend cheese
- 1/2 cup salsa
- 1 teaspoon chili powder
- 1/2 teaspoon cumin
- 1/4 teaspoon garlic powder
- Salt and pepper to taste
- 12 small corn tortillas
- Vegetable oil for frying
- Toppings (optional): sour cream, guacamole, additional salsa

1. In a medium bowl, mix together the shredded chicken, shredded cheese, salsa, chili powder, cumin, garlic powder, salt, and pepper until well combined.

2. Lay the corn tortillas out on a clean surface. Spoon about 2-3 tablespoons of the chicken and cheese mixture onto the center of each tortilla.

3. Carefully roll up each tortilla tightly around the filling to form a taquito.

4. In a large skillet or Dutch oven, heat about 1/2 inch of vegetable oil over medium-high heat.

5. Working in batches, fry the taquitos for 1-2 minutes per side until golden brown and crispy.

6. Transfer the fried taquitos to a paper towel-lined plate to drain any excess oil.

7. Serve the chicken and cheese taquitos warm, with your desired toppings like sour cream, guacamole, or additional salsa.

These taquitos are a fun and portable snack or appetizer that young teens are sure to love. The crispy tortilla shell and flavorful chicken and cheese filling make them irresistible. Enjoy!

Did you have fun cooking this dish?

 ◯   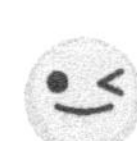 ◯

How would you rate this dish?

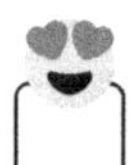 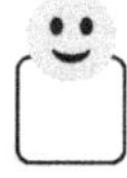 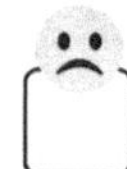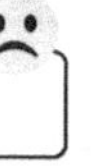 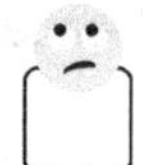 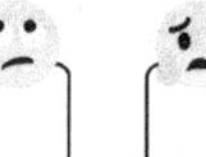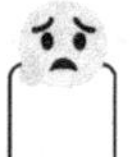

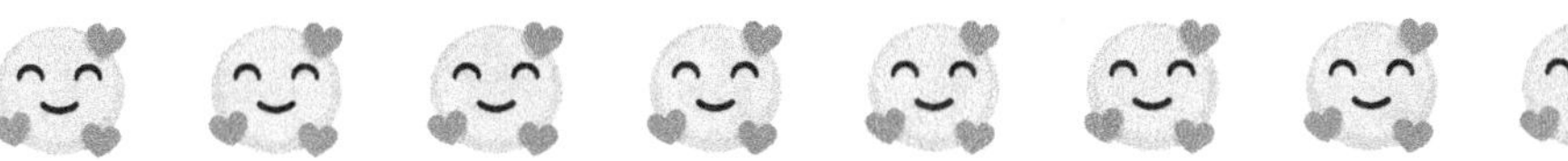

94. Loaded chili cheese dogs

 Prep Time : 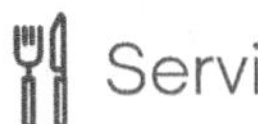 Cook Time : Servings :

Write 5 friends with whom you want to share this dish

....
....
....
....
....

Is this dish easy or difficult for you to make?

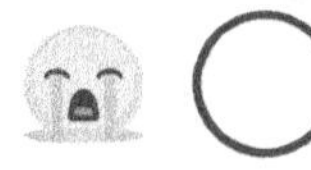 ◯   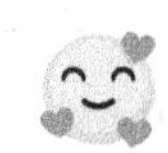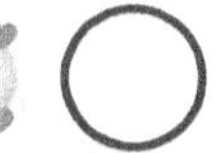 ◯

INGREDIENTS

- 8 hot dogs
- 8 hot dog buns
- 1 (15 oz) can chili with beans
- 1 cup shredded cheddar cheese
- 1/4 cup diced onion (optional)
- Toppings (optional): pickled jalapeños, sour cream, etc.

1. Preheat your oven to 350°F.

2. Place the hot dogs in a baking dish and bake for 10-12 minutes, until heated through.

3. Meanwhile, warm the chili in a small saucepan over medium heat, stirring occasionally.

4. Place the hot dog buns on a baking sheet and toast them in the oven for 2-3 minutes, until lightly golden.

5. Remove the hot dogs and buns from the oven.

6. Place each hot dog in a toasted bun. Top with a generous amount of the warm chili, followed by the shredded cheddar cheese and diced onion (if using).

7. Return the loaded chili cheese dogs to the oven for an additional 5 minutes, or until the cheese is melted and bubbly.

8. Serve the loaded chili cheese dogs hot, with any additional desired toppings like pickled jalapeños or sour cream.

These loaded chili cheese dogs are a fun and flavorful twist on a classic hot dog that young teens are sure to love. The combination of the savory chili, melted cheese, and crispy bun is simply irresistible. Enjoy!

Did you have fun cooking this dish?

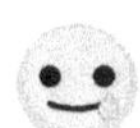 ◯   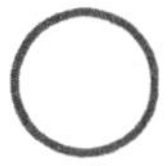 ◯

How would you rate this dish?

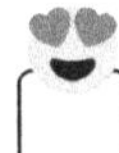 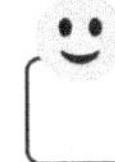  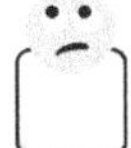 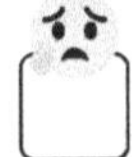

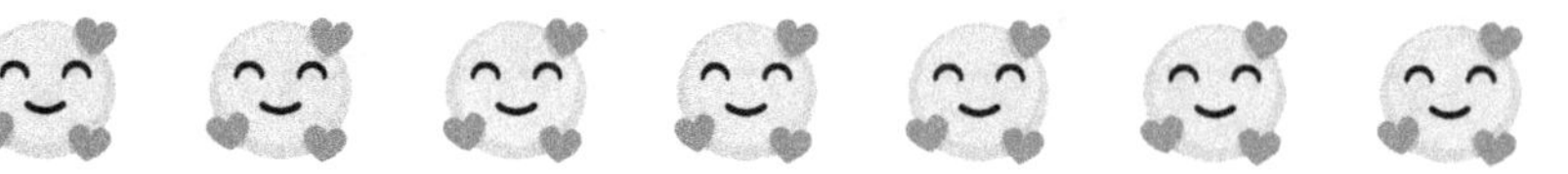

95. Beef and cheddar sliders

 Prep Time : 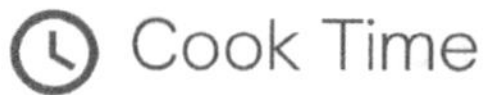 Cook Time :  Servings :

Write 5 friends with whom you want to share this dish

....
....
....
....
....

INGREDIENTS

- 1 lb ground beef
- 1 teaspoon garlic powder
- 1 teaspoon onion powder
- 1 teaspoon Worcestershire sauce
- Salt and pepper to taste
- 12 small slider buns or dinner rolls, split in half
- 6 slices cheddar cheese, cut in half

Is this dish easy or difficult for you to make?

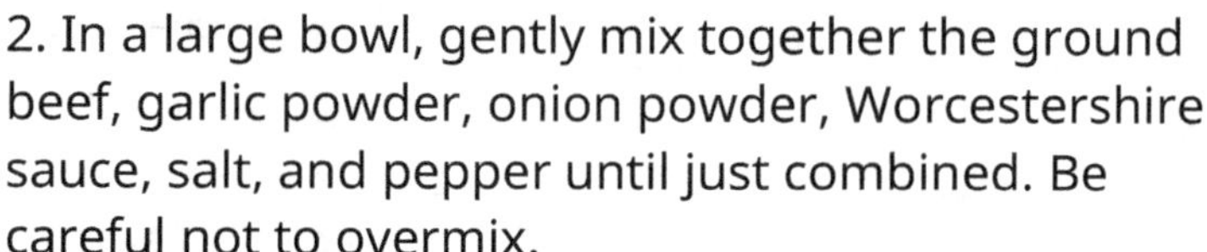

1. Preheat your oven to 375°F.

2. In a large bowl, gently mix together the ground beef, garlic powder, onion powder, Worcestershire sauce, salt, and pepper until just combined. Be careful not to overmix.

3. Divide the beef mixture into 12 equal portions and shape them into small patties, about 2-3 inches wide.

4. Heat a large skillet or griddle over medium-high heat. Cook the beef patties for 2-3 minutes per side, until they are lightly browned and cooked through.

5. Place the bottom halves of the slider buns on a baking sheet. Top each one with a beef patty and a half slice of cheddar cheese.

6. Bake the sliders in the preheated oven for 5-7 minutes, or until the cheese is melted and the buns are lightly toasted.

7. Remove the sliders from the oven and top with the remaining bun halves.

Serve the beef and cheddar sliders warm, with any additional toppings or condiments that your young teens might enjoy, such as pickles, ketchup, or mustard.

These mini burgers are the perfect size for young appetites and are sure to be a hit at any gathering or party. Enjoy!

Did you have fun cooking this dish?

 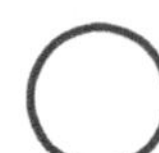    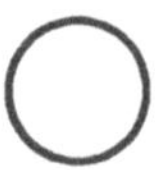

How would you rate this dish?

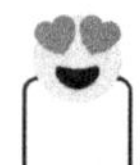  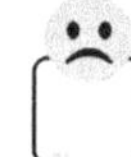  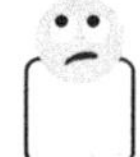 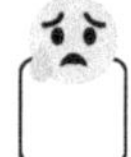

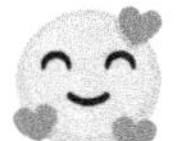  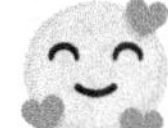 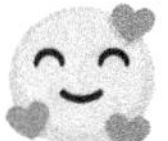 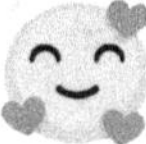 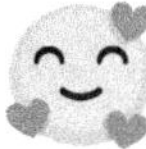 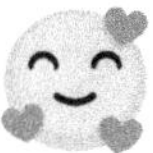 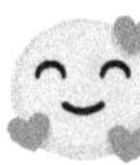 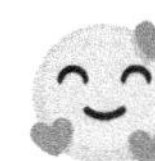 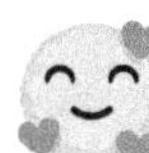

96. Buffalo chicken pizza

Let's do that and fill in the time here

Prep Time :

Cook Time :

Servings :

Write 5 friends with whom you want to share this dish

....

....

....

....

....

INGREDIENTS

- 1 lb boneless, skinless chicken breasts
- 1/2 cup buffalo sauce (such as Frank's RedHot)
- 1 pre-baked pizza crust or flatbread
- 1 cup shredded mozzarella cheese
- 1/4 cup crumbled blue cheese (optional)
- 2 tablespoons chopped fresh parsley (optional)

Is this dish easy or difficult for you to make?

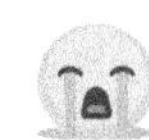 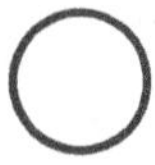 ◯   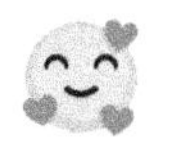 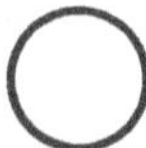 ◯

1. Preheat your oven to 400°F.

2. Place the chicken breasts in a baking dish and bake for 20-25 minutes, until cooked through. Allow to cool slightly, then shred the chicken using two forks.

3. In a bowl, mix the shredded chicken with the buffalo sauce until well coated.

4. Place the pre-baked pizza crust or flatbread on a baking sheet. Spread the buffalo chicken mixture evenly over the surface, leaving a small border around the edges.

5. Sprinkle the shredded mozzarella cheese over the top of the chicken.

6. If desired, crumble the blue cheese over the pizza as well.

7. Bake the buffalo chicken pizza in the preheated oven for 10-12 minutes, or until the cheese is melted and bubbly.

8. Remove the pizza from the oven and sprinkle with the chopped fresh parsley, if using.

9. Slice the pizza and serve it warm.

This buffalo chicken pizza is a fun and flavorful twist on a classic that young teens are sure to love. The spicy buffalo sauce, tender chicken, and melty cheese make for an irresistible combination. Enjoy!

Did you have fun cooking this dish?

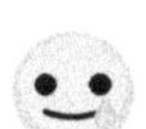 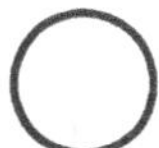 ◯    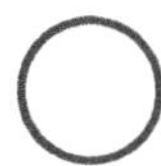 ◯

How would you rate this dish?

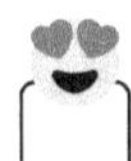 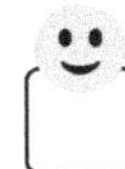 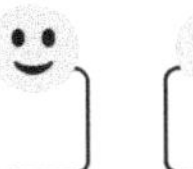 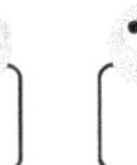 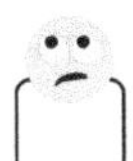 

97. Cheese-stuffed pretzels

 Prep Time : 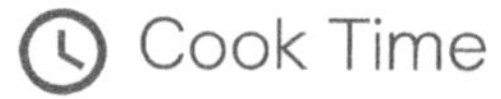 Cook Time : 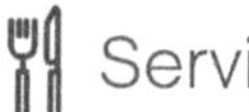 Servings :

Let's do that and fill in the time here

Write 5 friends with whom you want to share this dish ....

Is this dish easy or difficult for you to make?

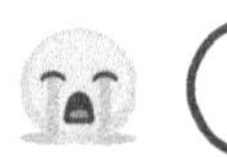 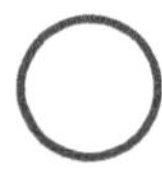 ◯    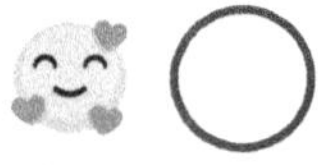 ◯

INGREDIENTS

- 1 package (16 oz) refrigerated pizza dough
- 4 oz cream cheese, softened
- 1/2 cup shredded cheddar cheese
- 1 egg, beaten with 1 tbsp water (for egg wash)
- Coarse sea salt or pretzel salt (optional)

For the Baking Soda Bath:
- 10 cups water
- 1/2 cup baking soda

1. Preheat your oven to 400°F. Line a baking sheet with parchment paper.

2. In a small bowl, mix together the softened cream cheese and shredded cheddar cheese until well combined.

3. Unroll the pizza dough and cut it into 8 equal pieces.

4. On a lightly floured surface, roll each piece of dough into a 6-inch rope.

5. Place a heaping tablespoon of the cheese mixture in the center of each dough rope. Fold the dough over the filling and pinch the seams to seal, forming a pretzel shape.

6. In a large pot, bring the 10 cups of water and 1/2 cup of baking soda to a boil.

7. Working in batches, carefully drop the stuffed pretzels into the boiling baking soda water for 30 seconds, then use a slotted spoon to transfer them to the prepared baking sheet.

8. Brush the tops of the pretzels with the beaten egg wash and sprinkle with coarse salt, if desired.

9. Bake the cheese-stuffed pretzels in the preheated oven for 12-15 minutes, until golden brown.

10. Serve the warm, gooey pretzels immediately.

These cheese-stuffed pretzels are a fun and tasty snack that young teens are sure to love. The melty cheese center is a delightful surprise in every bite!

Did you have fun cooking this dish?

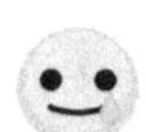 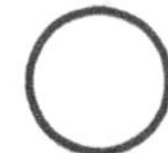 ◯   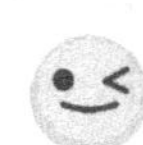 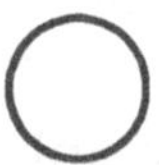 ◯

How would you rate this dish?

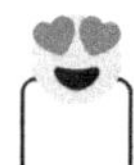 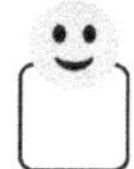 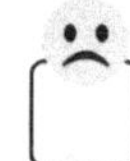 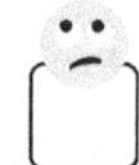 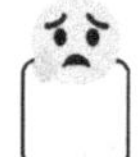

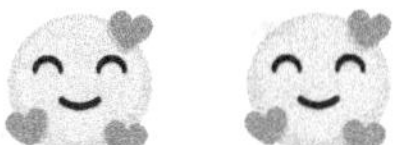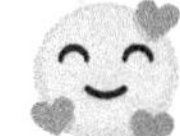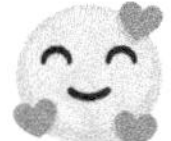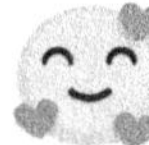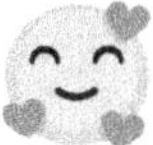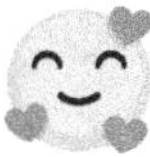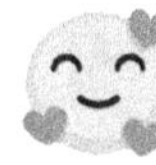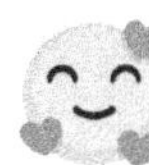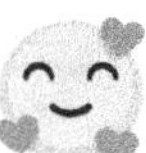

98. Chicken bacon ranch pizza

Prep Time :   Cook Time :   Servings :

Is this dish easy or difficult for you to make?

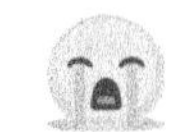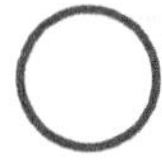 ◯   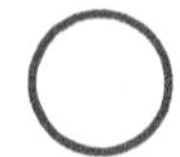 ◯

Write 5 friends with whom you want to share this dish

....

....

....

....

....

INGREDIENTS

- 1 lb ground beef
- 1 packet taco seasoning
- 1/2 cup water
- 1 (15 oz) can black beans, drained and rinsed
- 1 (12 oz) bag tortilla chips
- 2 cups shredded cheddar or Mexican blend cheese
- Toppings (optional): diced tomatoes, sliced jalapeños, sour cream, guacamole, etc.

1. Preheat your oven to 375°F.

2. In a large skillet, cook the ground beef over medium heat until browned and crumbled, about 5-7 minutes. Drain any excess fat.

3. Add the taco seasoning and water to the skillet. Stir and simmer for 2-3 minutes until the sauce thickens.

4. Stir in the drained and rinsed black beans.

5. Spread the tortilla chips out in a single layer on a large baking sheet or oven-safe platter.

6. Spoon the beef and bean mixture evenly over the chips, then sprinkle the shredded cheese on top.

7. Bake the nachos in the preheated oven for 5-7 minutes, or until the cheese is melted and bubbly.

8. Remove the nachos from the oven and top with any desired toppings like diced tomatoes, sliced jalapeños, sour cream, or guacamole.

Serve the beef and cheese nachos immediately, while the chips are still warm and crispy. This is a fun and easy-to-eat dish that young teens are sure to love!

Did you have fun cooking this dish?

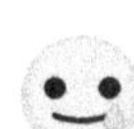 ◯   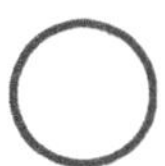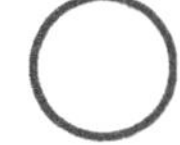 ◯

How would you rate this dish?

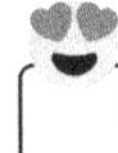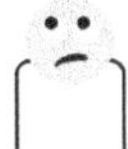

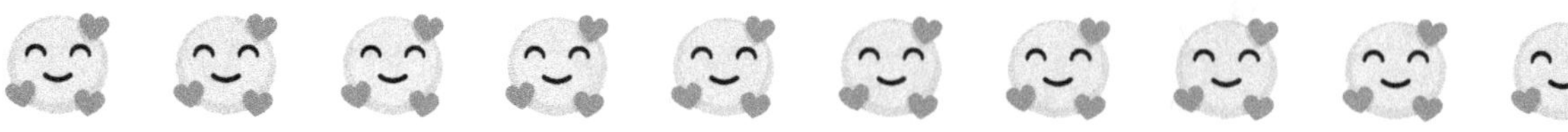

99. Beef and cheese nachos

Let's do that and fill in the time here

 Prep Time :   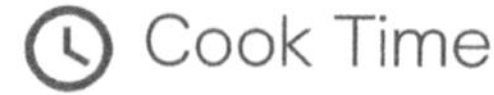 Cook Time :    Servings :

Write 5 friends with whom you want to share this dish

....

....

....

....

....

Is this dish easy or difficult for you to make?

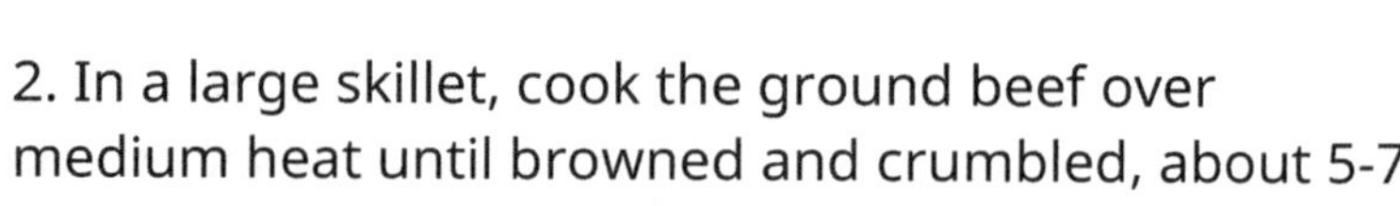

INGREDIENTS

- 1 lb ground beef
- 1 packet taco seasoning
- 1/2 cup water
- 1 (15 oz) can black beans, drained and rinsed
- 1 (12 oz) bag tortilla chips
- 2 cups shredded cheddar or Mexican blend cheese
- Toppings (optional): diced tomatoes, sliced jalapeños, sour cream, guacamole, etc.

1. Preheat your oven to 375°F.

2. In a large skillet, cook the ground beef over medium heat until browned and crumbled, about 5-7 minutes. Drain any excess fat.

3. Add the taco seasoning and water to the skillet. Stir and simmer for 2-3 minutes until the sauce thickens.

4. Stir in the drained and rinsed black beans.

5. Spread the tortilla chips out in a single layer on a large baking sheet or oven-safe platter.

6. Spoon the beef and bean mixture evenly over the chips, then sprinkle the shredded cheese on top.

7. Bake the nachos in the preheated oven for 5-7 minutes, or until the cheese is melted and bubbly.

8. Remove the nachos from the oven and top with any desired toppings like diced tomatoes, sliced jalapeños, sour cream, or guacamole.

Serve the beef and cheese nachos immediately, while the chips are still warm and crispy. This is a fun and easy-to-eat dish that everyone will love!

Did you have fun cooking this dish?

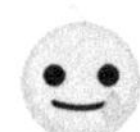 ◯    ◯

How would you rate this dish?

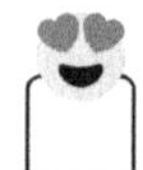 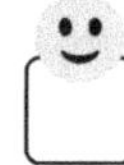  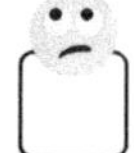 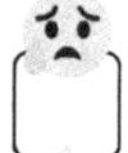

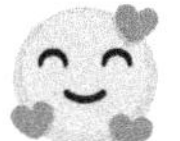 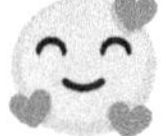 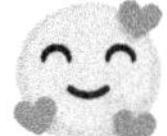 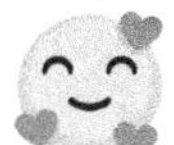 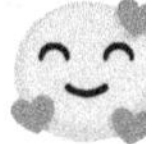 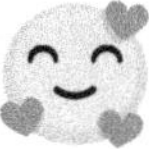 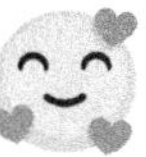 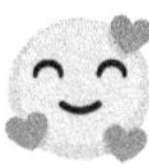  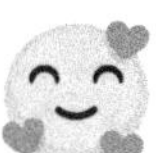

100. Loaded pizza fries

Let's do that and fill in the time here  Prep Time :    Cook Time :   Servings :

Write 5 friends with whom you want to share this dish

....

....

....

....

....

Is this dish easy or difficult for you to make?

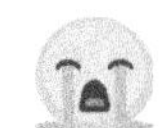 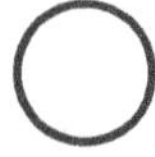 ◯   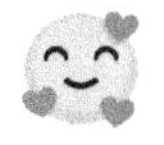 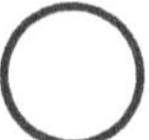 ◯

INGREDIENTS

- 1 lb frozen french fries
- 1 lb ground Italian sausage, casings removed
- 1 (15 oz) can pizza sauce
- 1 cup shredded mozzarella cheese
- 1/4 cup grated Parmesan cheese
- 1 teaspoon dried oregano
- Chopped fresh basil (optional)

1. Preheat your oven to 425°F. Spread the frozen french fries in a single layer on a large baking sheet.

2. Bake the fries for 20-25 minutes, flipping halfway, until golden brown and crispy.

3. While the fries are baking, cook the ground Italian sausage in a skillet over medium heat, breaking it up with a wooden spoon, until browned and cooked through, about 5-7 minutes. Drain any excess fat.

4. Remove the baked fries from the oven and top them with the cooked sausage.

5. Pour the pizza sauce evenly over the fries and sausage, then sprinkle the shredded mozzarella and grated Parmesan cheeses on top.

6. Return the loaded fries to the oven and bake for an additional 5-7 minutes, until the cheese is melted and bubbly.

7. Remove the loaded pizza fries from the oven and sprinkle with the dried oregano and chopped fresh basil (if using).

8. Serve the loaded pizza fries immediately, while hot and crispy.

These loaded pizza fries are a fun and delicious twist on classic french fries that young teens are sure to love. The combination of crispy fries, savory sausage, melted cheese, and pizza sauce is irresistible!

Did you have fun cooking this dish?

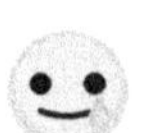 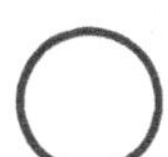 ◯    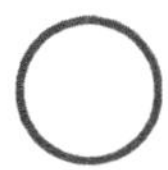 ◯

How would you rate this dish?

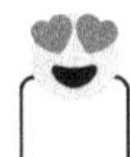 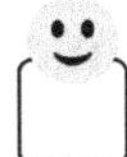 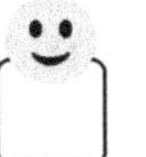  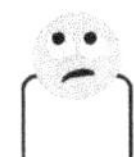 

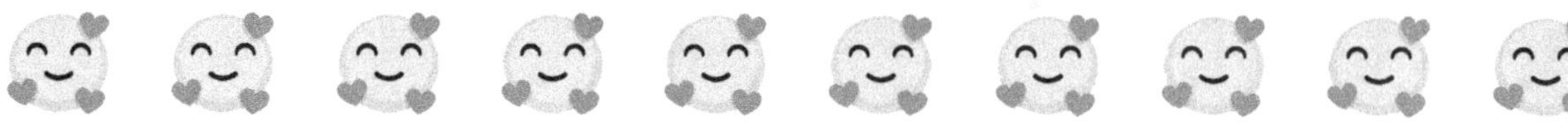

101. Chicken parmesan pasta

 Prep Time : 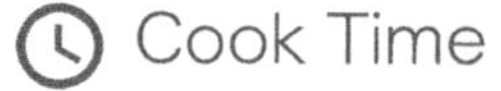 Cook Time : 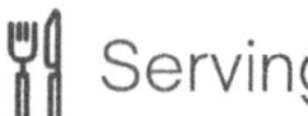 Servings :

Is this dish easy or difficult for you to make?

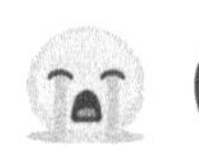 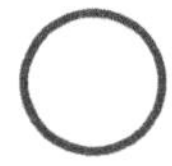 ◯   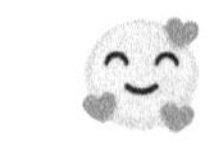 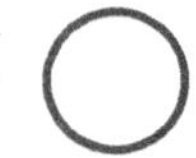 ◯

Write 5 friends with whom you want to share this dish

....

....

....

....

....

INGREDIENTS

- 4 boneless, skinless chicken breasts
- 1 cup all-purpose flour
- 2 eggs, beaten
- 1 cup breadcrumbs
- 1/2 cup grated Parmesan cheese
- 1 teaspoon dried oregano
- 1/2 teaspoon garlic powder
- Salt and pepper to taste
- 8 oz spaghetti or penne pasta
- 1 jar (24 oz) marinara sauce
- 1 cup shredded mozzarella cheese

1. Preheat your oven to 400°F.

2. Pound the chicken breasts between two sheets of plastic wrap or wax paper to an even 1/2-inch thickness.

3. Set up a breading station with the flour, beaten eggs, and a mixture of the breadcrumbs, Parmesan, oregano, garlic powder, salt, and pepper.

4. Dredge the chicken breasts in the flour, then dip them in the egg, and finally coat them in the breadcrumb mixture, pressing to adhere.

5. Place the breaded chicken on a baking sheet and bake for 20-25 minutes, until the chicken is cooked through and the breading is golden brown.

6. Meanwhile, cook the pasta according to the package instructions. Drain and set aside.

7. In a large baking dish, spread a layer of marinara sauce on the bottom. Place the baked chicken breasts on top and cover with the remaining marinara sauce.

8. Sprinkle the shredded mozzarella cheese over the top.

9. Bake the chicken parmesan for an additional 10-15 minutes, until the cheese is melted and bubbly. Serve the chicken parmesan over the cooked pasta.

This chicken parmesan pasta dish is a classic that young teens are sure to love. The crispy, breaded chicken paired with the flavorful marinara sauce and melted cheese is a winning combination. Enjoy!

Did you have fun cooking this dish?

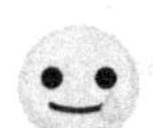 ◯    ◯

How would you rate this dish?

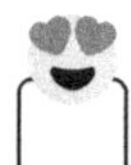 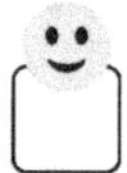 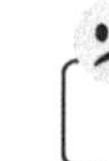 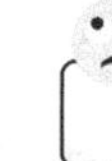 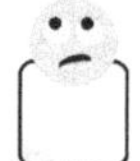 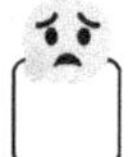

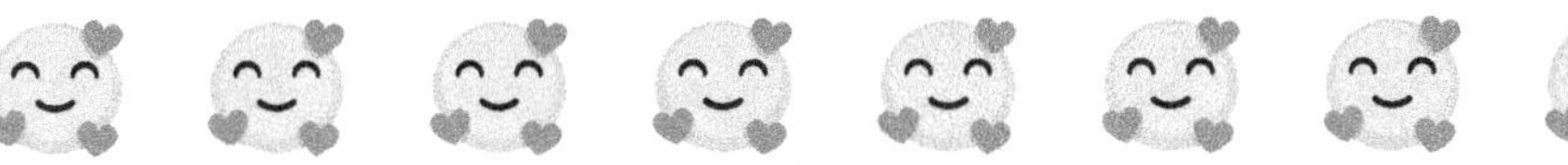

102. Beef and bean chalupa

Let's do that and fill in the time here

 Prep Time : 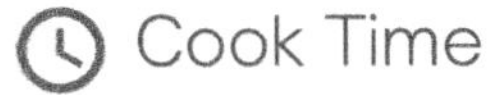 Cook Time : 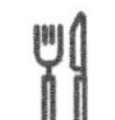 Servings :

Write 5 friends with whom you want to share this dish

....
....
....
....
....

Is this dish easy or difficult for you to make?

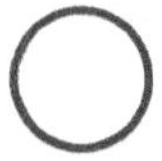 ◯   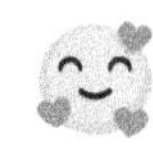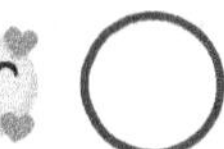 ◯

INGREDIENTS

- 1 lb ground beef
- 1 packet taco seasoning
- 1/2 cup water
- 1 (15 oz) can refried beans
- 8 tostada shells or chalupa shells
- 1 cup shredded lettuce
- 1 cup diced tomatoes
- 1 cup shredded cheddar cheese
- Toppings (optional): sour cream, salsa, guacamole, etc.

1. In a large skillet, cook the ground beef over medium heat until browned and crumbled, about 5-7 minutes. Drain any excess fat.

2. Add the taco seasoning and water to the skillet. Stir and simmer for 2-3 minutes until the sauce thickens.

3. Spread about 2-3 tablespoons of the refried beans onto each tostada or chalupa shell.

4. Top the refried beans with a heaping spoonful of the seasoned ground beef.

5. Sprinkle the shredded lettuce, diced tomatoes, and shredded cheddar cheese over the beef.

6. If desired, add any additional toppings like sour cream, salsa, or guacamole.

7. Serve the beef and bean chalupas immediately, while the shells are still crispy.

These chalupas are a fun and flavorful Mexican-inspired dish that young teens are sure to love. The combination of the crispy tostada shell, savory beef, creamy beans, and fresh toppings makes for a delicious and satisfying meal or snack.

Did you have fun cooking this dish?

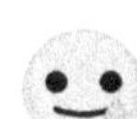 ◯   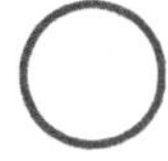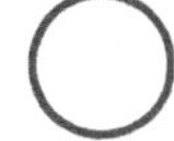 ◯

How would you rate this dish?

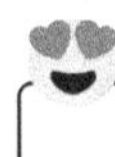 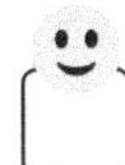  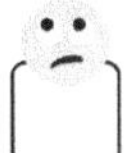 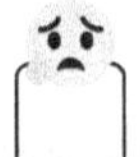

103. Cheesy breadsticks

 Prep Time : 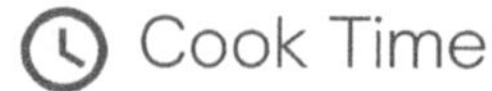 Cook Time : 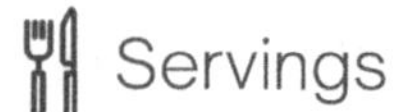 Servings :

Is this dish easy or difficult for you to make?

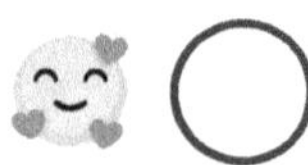 ◯   ◯

Write 5 friends with whom you want to share this dish

....

....

....

....

....

INGREDIENTS

- 1 lb pizza dough, store-bought or homemade
- 4 tablespoons unsalted butter, melted
- 1 teaspoon garlic powder
- 1 teaspoon dried oregano
- 1/2 teaspoon salt
- 2 cups shredded mozzarella cheese
- 1/4 cup grated Parmesan cheese
- Marinara sauce or ranch dressing, for dipping (optional)

1. Preheat your oven to 400°F. Line a large baking sheet with parchment paper.

2. On a lightly floured surface, roll or stretch the pizza dough into a large rectangle, about 12x8 inches.

3. Transfer the dough to the prepared baking sheet.

4. In a small bowl, mix together the melted butter, garlic powder, dried oregano, and salt.

5. Brush the butter mixture evenly over the surface of the dough.

6. Sprinkle the shredded mozzarella and grated Parmesan cheeses over the top.

7. Use a pizza cutter or sharp knife to slice the dough into 1-inch wide strips, leaving them attached at the base.

8. Bake the cheesy breadsticks in the preheated oven for 15-18 minutes, or until the cheese is melted and bubbly and the edges are golden brown.

9. Remove the breadsticks from the oven and let them cool for a few minutes.

10. Serve the warm cheesy breadsticks with marinara sauce or ranch dressing for dipping, if desired.

These cheesy breadsticks are a fun and easy-to-eat snack or appetizer that young teens are sure to love. The gooey, melted cheese and crispy edges make them irresistible!

Did you have fun cooking this dish?

 ◯   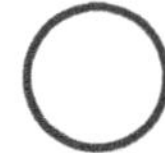 ◯

How would you rate this dish?

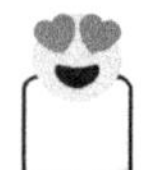 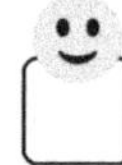  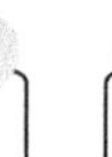 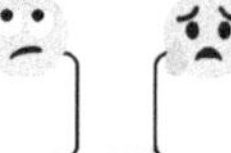

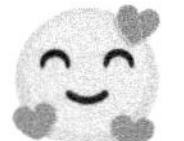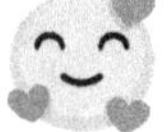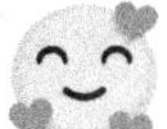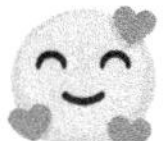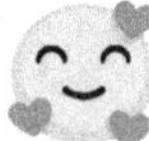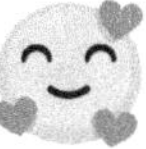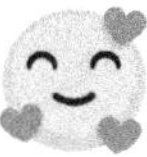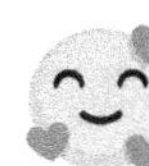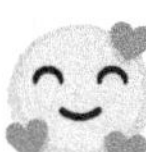

104. BBQ chicken nachos

Let's do that and fill in the time here

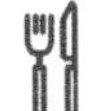 Prep Time :   Cook Time :   Servings :

Write 5 friends with whom you want to share this dish
....
....
....
....
....

Is this dish easy or difficult for you to make?

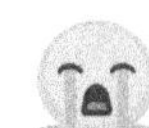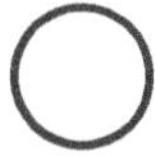 ◯   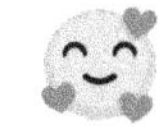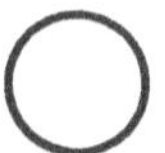 ◯

INGREDIENTS

- 1 lb boneless, skinless chicken breasts
- 1 cup barbecue sauce, divided
- 1 (12 oz) bag tortilla chips
- 2 cups shredded cheddar or Mexican blend cheese
- 1/2 cup diced red onion
- 2 tablespoons chopped fresh cilantro (optional)
- Toppings (optional): sour cream, jalapeños, etc.

1. Preheat your oven to 400°F.

2. Place the chicken breasts in a baking dish and brush them with 1/4 cup of the barbecue sauce. Bake for 20-25 minutes, until the chicken is cooked through. Allow to cool slightly, then shred the chicken using two forks.

3. In a bowl, mix the shredded chicken with the remaining 3/4 cup of barbecue sauce.

4. Spread the tortilla chips out in a single layer on a large baking sheet or oven-safe platter.

5. Spoon the BBQ chicken mixture evenly over the chips, then sprinkle the shredded cheese on top.

6. Bake the nachos in the preheated oven for 5-7 minutes, or until the cheese is melted and bubbly.

7. Remove the nachos from the oven and top with the diced red onion and chopped cilantro (if using).

8. Serve the BBQ chicken nachos immediately, with any additional desired toppings like sour cream or jalapeños.

These BBQ chicken nachos are a fun and flavorful twist on a classic that young teens are sure to love. The combination of the sweet and tangy barbecue sauce, tender chicken, and melty cheese is irresistible!

Did you have fun cooking this dish?

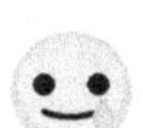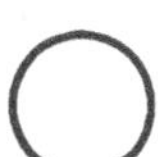 ◯   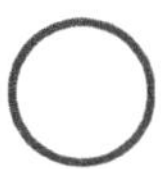 ◯

How would you rate this dish?

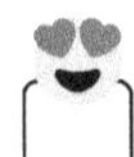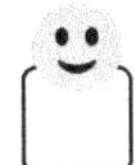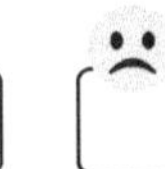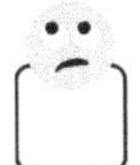

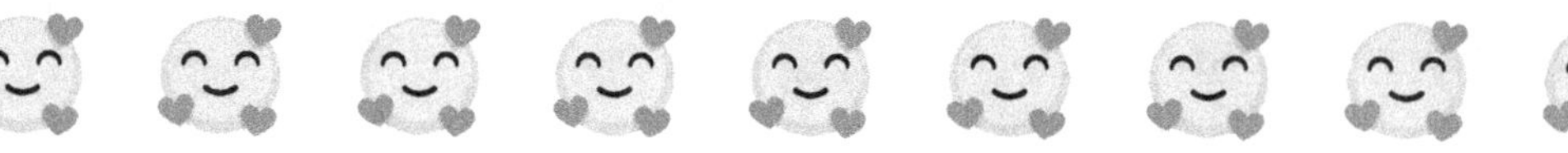

105. Beef and cheese empanadas

 Prep Time : 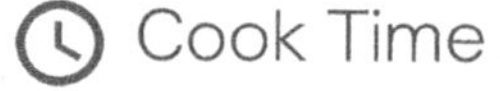 Cook Time : 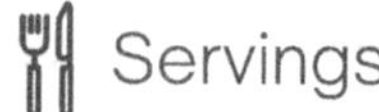 Servings :

Write 5 friends with whom you want to share this dish

....
....
....
....
....

Is this dish easy or difficult for you to make?

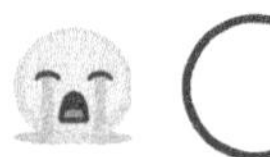 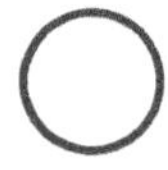 ◯   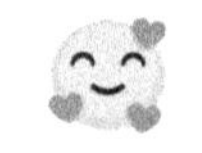 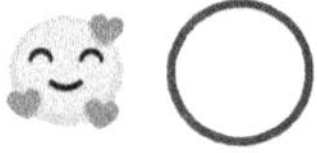 ◯

INGREDIENTS

- 1 lb ground beef
- 1 onion, diced
- 2 cloves garlic, minced
- 1 teaspoon cumin
- 1 teaspoon chili powder
- 1/2 teaspoon oregano
- Salt and pepper to taste
- 1 cup shredded cheddar or Monterey Jack cheese
- 1 package (14 oz) refrigerated pie crusts or empanada discs
- 1 egg, beaten with 1 tablespoon water (for egg wash)

1. Preheat your oven to 400°F. Line a baking sheet with parchment paper.

2. In a skillet over medium heat, cook the ground beef until browned and crumbled, 5-7 minutes. Drain any excess fat.

3. Add the diced onion and minced garlic to the skillet. Cook for 2-3 minutes until the onion is translucent.

4. Stir in the cumin, chili powder, oregano, salt, and pepper. Cook for 1 minute to toast the spices.

5. Remove the skillet from heat and stir in the shredded cheese until well combined. Allow the filling to cool slightly.

6. Unroll the pie crusts or empanada discs and cut each one into 4 equal wedges.

7. Place a heaping tablespoon of the beef and cheese filling onto the center of each wedge.

8. Fold the dough over the filling to create a half-moon shape and crimp the edges with a fork to seal.

9. Place the empanadas on the prepared baking sheet. Brush the tops with the egg wash.

10. Bake the empanadas for 18-22 minutes, until the crust is golden brown.

11. Serve the warm beef and cheese empanadas with your favorite dipping sauces, like salsa or guacamole.

Did you have fun cooking this dish?

 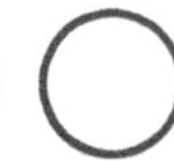 ◯    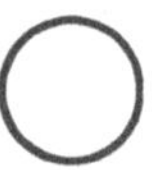 ◯

How would you rate this dish?

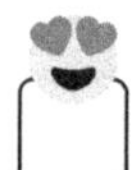 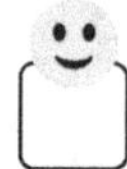  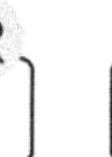 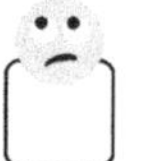 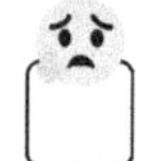

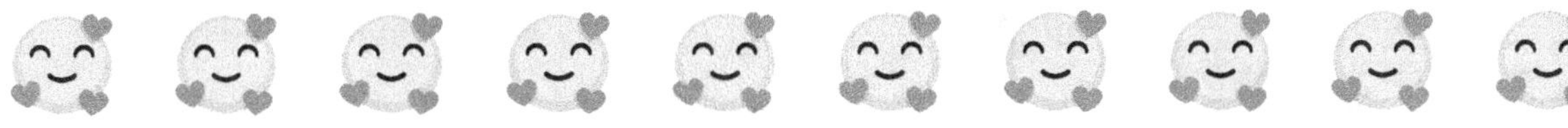

106. Buffalo chicken mac and cheese

 Prep Time : 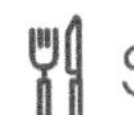 Cook Time : Servings :

Write 5 friends with whom you want to share this dish

....

....

....

....

....

Is this dish easy or difficult for you to make?

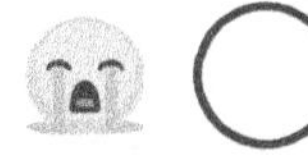 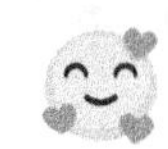 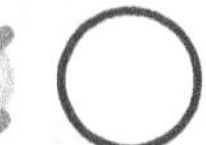 ○   ○

INGREDIENTS

- 8 oz elbow macaroni
- 2 boneless, skinless chicken breasts
- 1/2 cup buffalo sauce (such as Frank's RedHot)
- 2 tablespoons unsalted butter
- 2 tablespoons all-purpose flour
- 2 cups milk
- 2 cups shredded cheddar cheese
- 1/4 cup crumbled blue cheese (optional)
- Salt and pepper to taste
- Chopped fresh parsley for garnish (optional)

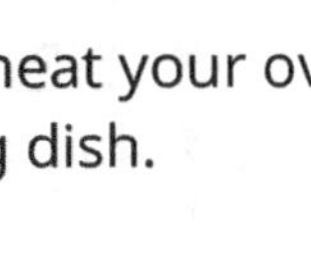

1. Preheat your oven to 375°F. Grease a 9x13 inch baking dish.

2. Cook the macaroni according to package instructions. Drain and set aside.

3. Place the chicken breasts in a baking dish and bake for 20-25 minutes, until cooked through. Allow to cool slightly, then shred the chicken using two forks.

4. In a large saucepan, melt the butter over medium heat. Whisk in the flour and cook for 1 minute.

5. Gradually whisk in the milk and cook, stirring constantly, until the sauce thickens, about 5 minutes.

6. Remove the sauce from heat and stir in the shredded cheddar cheese until melted and smooth.

7. Add the cooked macaroni, shredded chicken, and buffalo sauce to the cheese sauce. Stir to combine.

8. Transfer the buffalo chicken mac and cheese to the prepared baking dish. Sprinkle the crumbled blue cheese on top, if using.

9. Bake for 20-25 minutes, until hot and bubbly.

10. Remove from the oven and garnish with chopped fresh parsley, if desired.

Serve this buffalo chicken mac and cheese warm. The spicy buffalo flavor combined with the creamy, cheesy pasta is sure to be a hit with young teens!

Did you have fun cooking this dish?

  ○    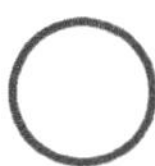 ○

How would you rate this dish?

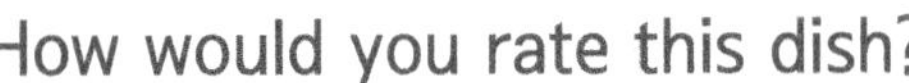

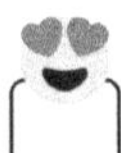 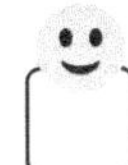 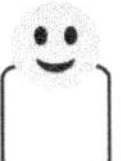  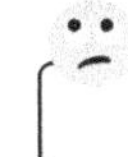 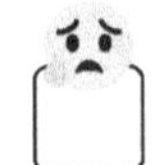

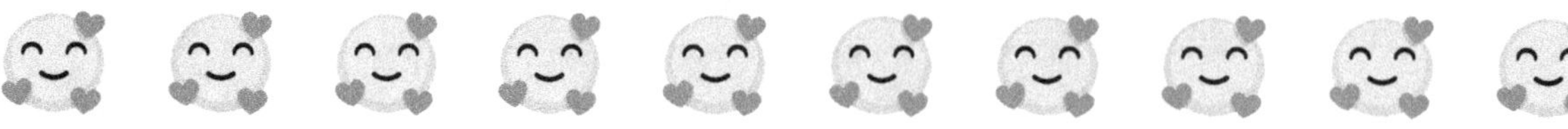

107. Loaded cheeseburger

 *Let's do that and fill in the time here* 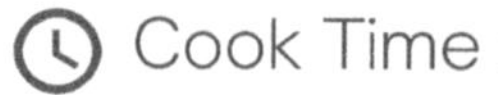 Prep Time :  Cook Time : 🍴 Servings :

Write 5 friends with whom you want to share this dish

....

....

....

....

....

Is this dish easy or difficult for you to make?

😭 ◯   😊 ◯

INGREDIENTS

- 1 lb ground beef
- 1 teaspoon salt
- 1/2 teaspoon black pepper
- 4 hamburger buns, split in half
- 4 slices cheddar cheese
- 4 slices bacon, cooked until crispy
- 1 tomato, sliced
- 1 cup shredded lettuce
- Condiments (optional): ketchup, mustard, mayonnaise, pickles, etc.

1. Preheat your grill or a large skillet over medium-high heat.

2. In a bowl, gently mix the ground beef with the salt and pepper until just combined. Divide the mixture into 4 equal portions and shape them into patties, about 4-5 inches wide and 1/2 inch thick.

3. Grill or cook the patties in the skillet for 3-4 minutes per side, or until they reach your desired level of doneness.

4. During the last minute of cooking, top each patty with a slice of cheddar cheese to melt.

5. Place the cheeseburger patties on the bottom buns. Top each one with 1-2 slices of crispy bacon, a tomato slice, and a handful of shredded lettuce.

6. Add any desired condiments to the top buns and place them on the burgers.

7. Serve the loaded cheeseburgers immediately, while the cheese is still melted.

These loaded cheeseburgers are sure to be a hit with young teens. The combination of the juicy beef patty, melted cheese, crispy bacon, and fresh toppings makes for a delicious and satisfying burger that they'll love. Enjoy!

Did you have fun cooking this dish?

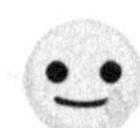 ◯  ◯

How would you rate this dish?

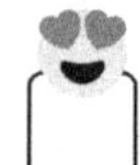 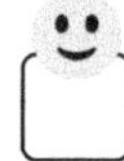  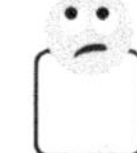 

  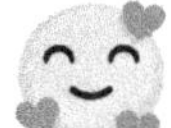 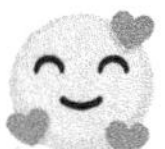 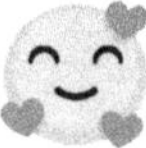 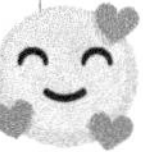 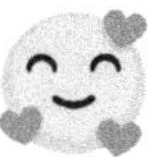 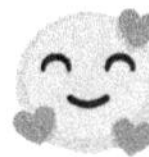 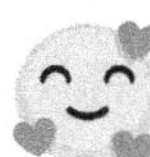 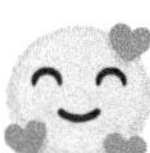

108. Chicken and waffle sliders

 Prep Time :   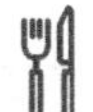 Cook Time :   Servings :

Write 5 friends with whom you want to share this dish

....

....

....

....

....

INGREDIENTS

- 8 frozen mini waffles
- 4 breaded and fried chicken tenders
- 4 slices cheddar cheese
- 2 tbsp maple syrup
- 2 tbsp butter, melted

Is this dish easy or difficult for you to make?

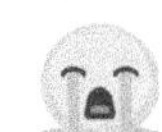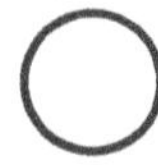 ◯   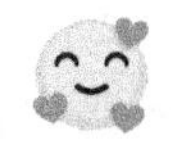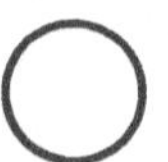 ◯

1. Preheat oven to 350°F. Place the frozen mini waffles on a baking sheet and bake for 5-7 minutes until warmed through.

2. While the waffles are warming, prepare the chicken tenders according to package instructions. Once cooked, cut each tender in half to create 8 slider-sized pieces.

3. Place a slice of cheddar cheese on 4 of the waffles. Top each cheese-topped waffle with a piece of chicken tender.

4. Brush the remaining 4 waffles with the melted butter.

5. Drizzle the maple syrup over the chicken tenders.

6. Close the sliders by placing the buttered waffles on top of the chicken and cheese.

7. Serve the chicken and waffle sliders warm.

Enjoy these fun and tasty chicken and waffle slider bites! The combination of the crispy chicken, sweet waffles, and maple syrup is delicious.

Did you have fun cooking this dish?

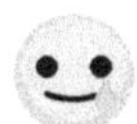 ◯   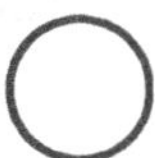 ◯

How would you rate this dish?

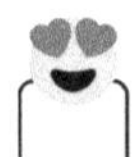 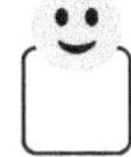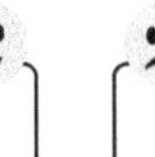 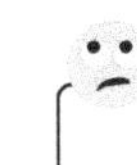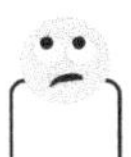 

109. Beef and cheese stuffed peppers

 Prep Time : 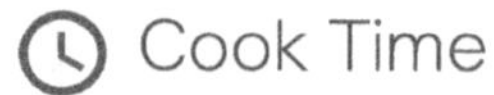 Cook Time :  Servings :

Is this dish easy or difficult for you to make?

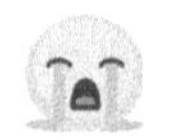 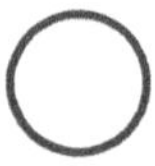 ◯    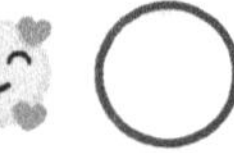 ◯

Write 5 friends with whom you want to share this dish

INGREDIENTS

- 6 bell peppers (any color), halved lengthwise and seeds removed
- 1 lb ground beef
- 1 onion, diced
- 2 cloves garlic, minced
- 1 cup cooked rice
- 1 (15 oz) can tomato sauce
- 1 teaspoon dried oregano
- 1/2 teaspoon chili powder
- Salt and pepper to taste
- 1 cup shredded cheddar or Monterey Jack cheese

1. Preheat your oven to 375°F. Arrange the bell pepper halves in a baking dish.

2. In a skillet over medium heat, cook the ground beef until browned and crumbled, 5-7 minutes. Drain any excess fat.

3. Add the diced onion and minced garlic to the skillet. Cook for 2-3 minutes until the onion is translucent.

4. Stir in the cooked rice, tomato sauce, oregano, chili powder, salt, and pepper. Cook for 2-3 minutes to allow the flavors to meld.

5. Spoon the beef and rice mixture evenly into the bell pepper halves, packing it in gently.

6. Sprinkle the shredded cheese over the top of the stuffed peppers.

7. Bake the stuffed peppers in the preheated oven for 20-25 minutes, until the peppers are tender and the cheese is melted and bubbly.

8. Remove the stuffed peppers from the oven and serve warm.

These beef and cheese stuffed peppers are a delicious and nutritious meal that young teens are sure to enjoy. The savory beef and rice filling paired with the sweet bell peppers and melted cheese makes for a winning combination.

Did you have fun cooking this dish?

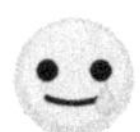 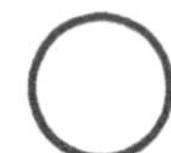 ◯    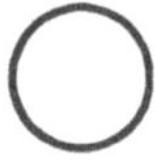 ◯

How would you rate this dish?

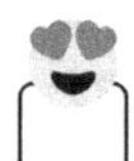 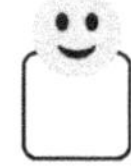  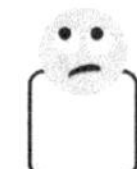 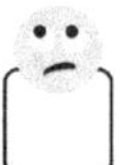 

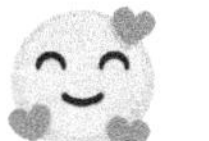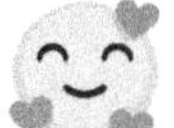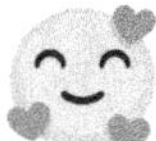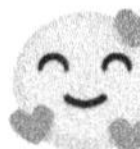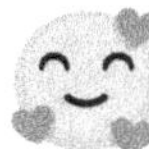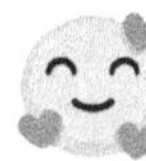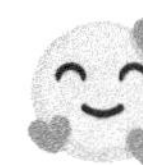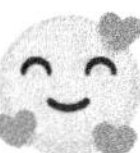

110. Cheesy garlic chicken

Let's do that and fill in the time here

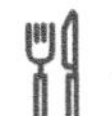 Prep Time :　　　Cook Time :　　　Servings :

Write 5 friends with whom you want to share this dish

....

....

....

....

....

Is this dish easy or difficult for you to make?

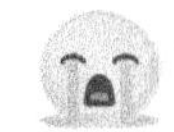 ◯　　　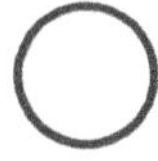 ◯

INGREDIENTS

- 4 boneless, skinless chicken breasts
- 1/2 cup grated Parmesan cheese
- 1/2 cup shredded mozzarella cheese
- 3 cloves garlic, minced
- 2 tablespoons olive oil
- 1 teaspoon dried oregano
- 1/2 teaspoon salt
- 1/4 teaspoon black pepper

1. Preheat your oven to 400°F. Grease a 9x13 inch baking dish.

2. In a small bowl, mix together the Parmesan cheese, mozzarella cheese, minced garlic, oregano, salt, and pepper.

3. Place the chicken breasts in the prepared baking dish. Drizzle the olive oil over the top of the chicken.

4. Evenly sprinkle the cheese and garlic mixture over the chicken breasts, pressing it gently to adhere.

5. Bake the cheesy garlic chicken in the preheated oven for 25-30 minutes, until the chicken is cooked through and the cheese is melted and bubbly.

6. Remove the chicken from the oven and let it rest for 5 minutes before serving.

Serve the cheesy garlic chicken warm, with any desired sides like roasted vegetables or mashed potatoes. The combination of the tender, juicy chicken, melted cheeses, and savory garlic makes this dish irresistible.

This recipe is simple to prepare but full of flavor, making it a great option for young teens and families alike. Enjoy!

Did you have fun cooking this dish?

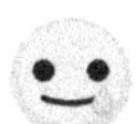  ◯　　　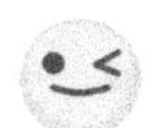 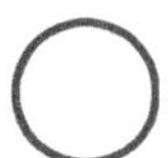 ◯

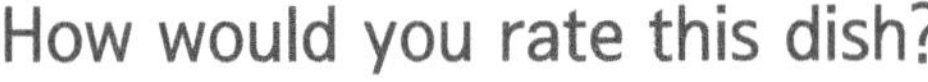

How would you rate this dish?

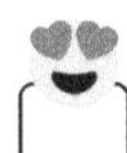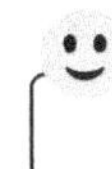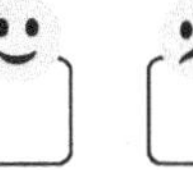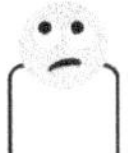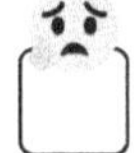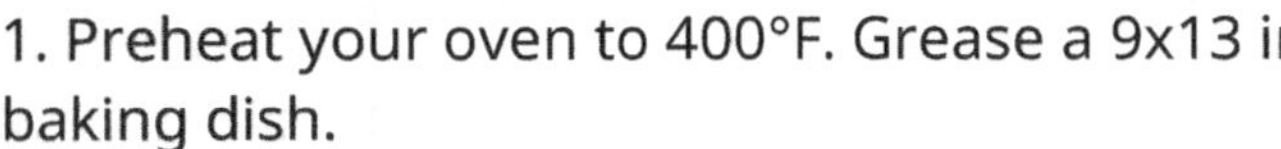

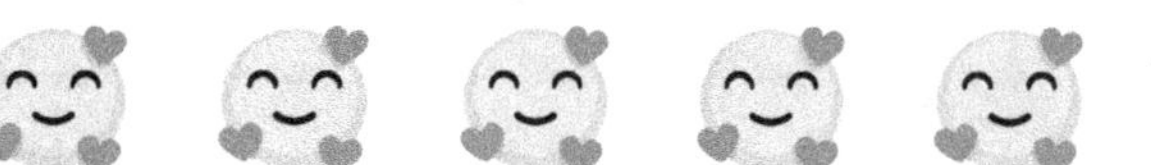

111. BBQ pulled pork nachos

Let's do that and fill in the time here   Prep Time :   Cook Time :   Servings :

Write 5 friends with whom you want to share this dish

....

....

....

....

....

Is this dish easy or difficult for you to make?

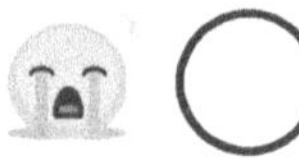 ◯   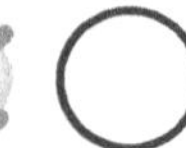 ◯

INGREDIENTS

- 1 lb pulled pork, store-bought or homemade
- 1 cup barbecue sauce
- 1 (12 oz) bag tortilla chips
- 2 cups shredded cheddar or Mexican blend cheese
- 1/2 cup diced red onion
- 1/4 cup sliced pickled jalapeños (optional)
- 2 tablespoons chopped fresh cilantro (optional)
- Sour cream, for serving (optional)

1. In a medium saucepan, combine the pulled pork and barbecue sauce. Heat over medium, stirring occasionally, until warmed through, about 5 minutes.

2. Preheat your oven to 400°F. Spread the tortilla chips out in a single layer on a large baking sheet or oven-safe platter.

3. Spoon the BBQ pulled pork evenly over the tortilla chips, making sure to cover them well.

4. Sprinkle the shredded cheese over the top of the pork.

5. Bake the nachos in the preheated oven for 5-7 minutes, or until the cheese is melted and bubbly.

6. Remove the nachos from the oven and top with the diced red onion, sliced jalapeños (if using), and chopped cilantro (if using).

7. Serve the BBQ pulled pork nachos immediately, with sour cream on the side for dipping, if desired.

These BBQ pulled pork nachos are a delicious and satisfying snack or meal. The tender, saucy pork, melted cheese, and crunchy chips make for an irresistible combination. Enjoy!

Did you have fun cooking this dish?

 ◯    ◯

How would you rate this dish?

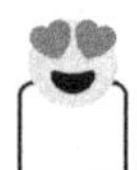 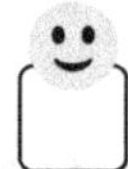 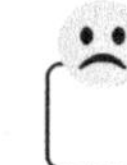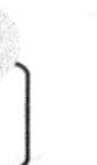 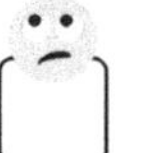 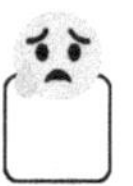

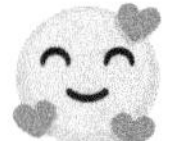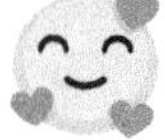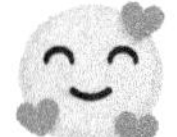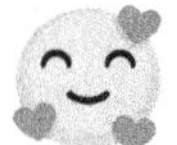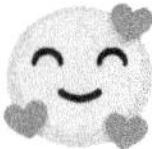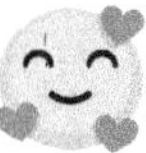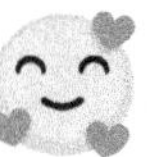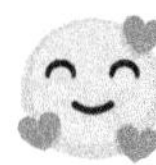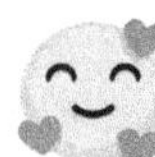

112. Beef and bean burrito bowl

Let's do that and fill in the time here  Prep Time :   Cook Time :   Servings :

Write 5 friends with whom you want to share this dish

INGREDIENTS

- 1 lb ground beef
- 1 packet taco seasoning
- 1/2 cup water
- 1 (15 oz) can black beans, drained and rinsed
- 2 cups cooked rice
- 1 cup shredded lettuce
- 1 cup diced tomatoes
- 1 cup shredded cheddar cheese
- Toppings (optional): sour cream, salsa, guacamole, etc.

Is this dish easy or difficult for you to make?

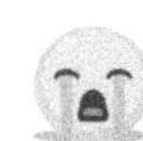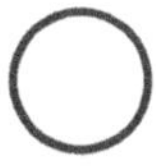 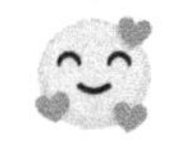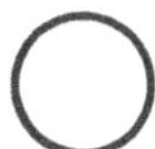

1. In a large skillet, cook the ground beef over medium heat until browned and crumbled, about 5-7 minutes. Drain any excess fat.

2. Add the taco seasoning and water to the skillet. Stir and simmer for 2-3 minutes until the sauce thickens.

3. Stir in the drained and rinsed black beans and cook for an additional 2-3 minutes.

4. Divide the cooked rice between 4 bowls.

5. Top the rice with the beef and bean mixture, shredded lettuce, diced tomatoes, and shredded cheddar cheese.

6. If desired, add any additional toppings like sour cream, salsa, or guacamole.

This beef and bean burrito bowl is a delicious and customizable meal that's perfect for young teens. The combination of the seasoned ground beef, creamy beans, fluffy rice, and fresh toppings makes for a satisfying and flavorful dish. Enjoy!

Did you have fun cooking this dish?

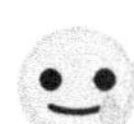 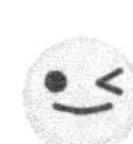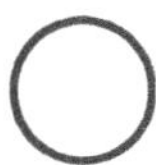

How would you rate this dish?

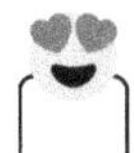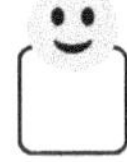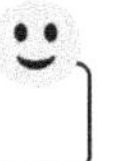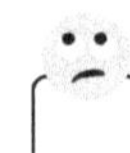

113. Chicken parmesan sliders

 Prep Time : 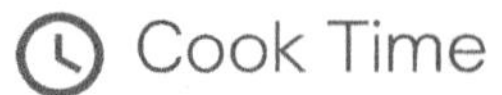  Cook Time : Servings :

Write 5 friends with whom you want to share this dish ....

Is this dish easy or difficult for you to make?

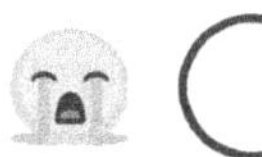 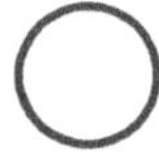 ◯ 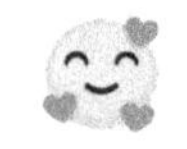 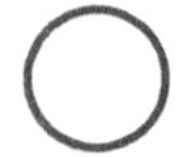 ◯

INGREDIENTS

- 1 lb boneless, skinless chicken breasts
- 1 cup all-purpose flour
- 2 eggs, beaten
- 1 cup breadcrumbs
- 1/2 cup grated Parmesan cheese
- 1 teaspoon dried oregano
- 1/2 teaspoon garlic powder
- Salt and pepper to taste
- 12 small slider buns or dinner rolls
- 1 cup marinara sauce
- 1 cup shredded mozzarella cheese

1. Preheat your oven to 400°F.

2. Pound the chicken breasts between two sheets of plastic wrap or wax paper to an even 1/4-inch thickness.

3. Set up a breading station with the flour, beaten eggs, and a mixture of the breadcrumbs, Parmesan, oregano, garlic powder, salt, and pepper.

4. Dredge the chicken in the flour, then dip in the egg, and finally coat in the breadcrumb mixture, pressing to adhere.

5. Place the breaded chicken on a baking sheet and bake for 15-18 minutes, until the chicken is cooked through and the breading is golden brown.

6. Remove the chicken from the oven and cut each breast into 6 equal slider-sized pieces.

7. Place the bottom halves of the slider buns on a baking sheet. Top each one with a piece of the chicken parmesan.

8. Spoon a tablespoon of marinara sauce over the chicken, then sprinkle the shredded mozzarella cheese on top.

9. Bake the chicken parmesan sliders in the preheated oven for 5-7 minutes, or until the cheese is melted and bubbly.

10. Remove the sliders from the oven and top with the remaining bun halves.

Did you have fun cooking this dish?

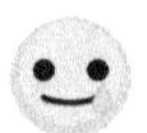  ◯  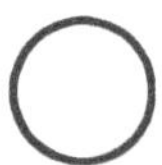 ◯

How would you rate this dish?

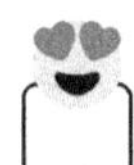 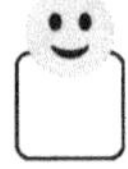 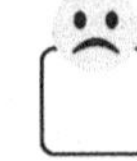 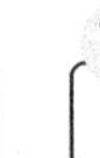 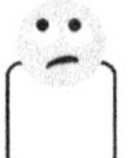 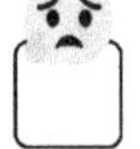

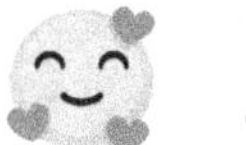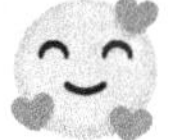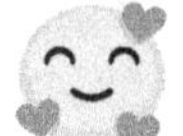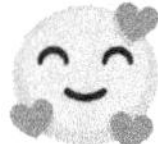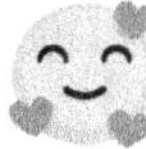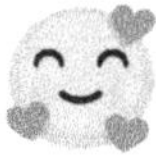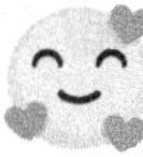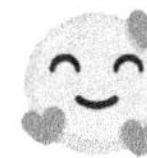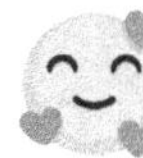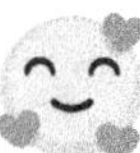

114. Loaded potato wedges

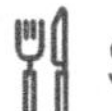 Prep Time :   Cook Time :   Servings :

Write 5 friends with whom you want to share this dish

....

....

....

....

....

INGREDIENTS

- 3 lbs russet potatoes, cut into 1/2-inch thick wedges
- 2 tablespoons olive oil
- 1 teaspoon salt
- 1/2 teaspoon black pepper
- 1 cup shredded cheddar cheese
- 6 slices bacon, cooked and crumbled
- 1/2 cup sour cream
- 2 tablespoons chopped fresh chives (optional)

Is this dish easy or difficult for you to make?

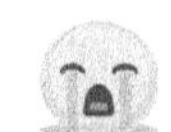 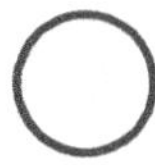 ◯   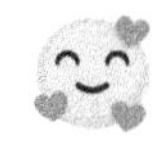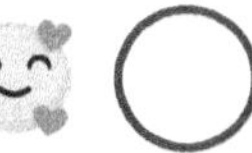 ◯

1. Preheat your oven to 400°F. Line a large baking sheet with parchment paper.

2. In a large bowl, toss the potato wedges with the olive oil, salt, and pepper until evenly coated.

3. Spread the seasoned potato wedges in a single layer on the prepared baking sheet.

4. Bake the potato wedges for 25-30 minutes, flipping halfway, until golden brown and crispy.

5. Remove the baked potato wedges from the oven and top them with the shredded cheddar cheese and crumbled bacon.

6. Return the loaded potato wedges to the oven for an additional 5 minutes, until the cheese is melted.

7. Transfer the loaded potato wedges to a serving platter or plate. Dollop the sour cream over the top and sprinkle with the chopped chives, if using.

8. Serve the loaded potato wedges warm, with any additional toppings or dipping sauces on the side.

These loaded potato wedges are a delicious and satisfying snack or side dish. The crispy baked potatoes, melted cheese, crispy bacon, and cool sour cream make for an irresistible combination. Enjoy!

Did you have fun cooking this dish?

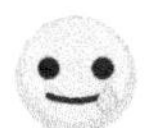 ◯   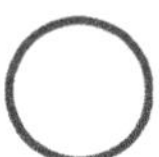 ◯

How would you rate this dish?

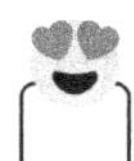 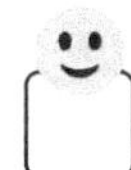 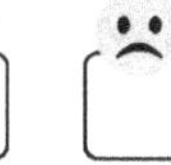 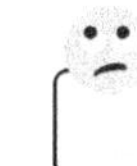 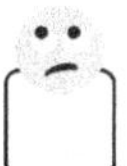 

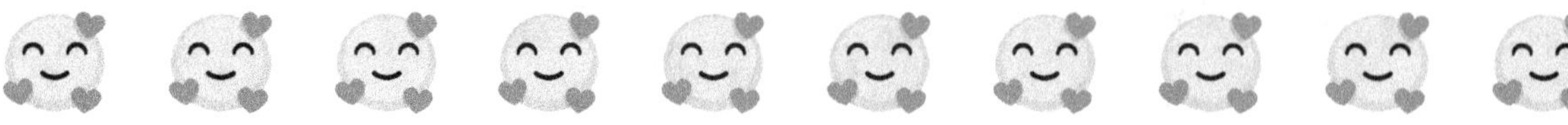

115. Beef and cheese stuffed shells

 *Let's do that and fill in the time here* **Prep Time :**   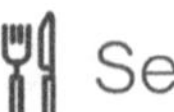 Cook Time :   Servings :

Write 5 friends with whom you want to share this dish ....

INGREDIENTS

- 12 oz jumbo pasta shells
- 1 lb ground beef
- 1 onion, diced
- 3 cloves garlic, minced
- 1 (15 oz) can tomato sauce
- 1 teaspoon dried oregano
- 1/2 teaspoon salt
- 1/4 teaspoon black pepper
- 1 (15 oz) container ricotta cheese
- 2 cups shredded mozzarella cheese, divided
- 1/2 cup grated Parmesan cheese
- 1 egg, lightly beaten

Did you have fun cooking this dish?

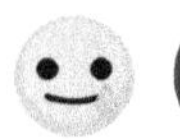 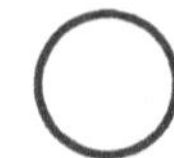 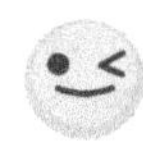 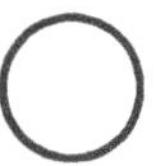

How would you rate this dish?

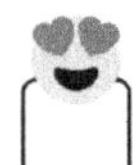 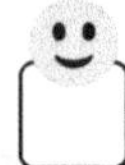  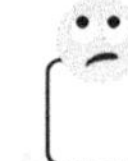 

Is this dish easy or difficult for you to make?

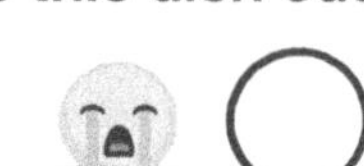 ○   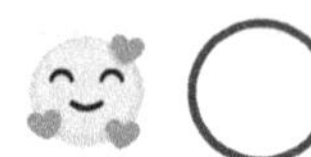 ○

1. Preheat your oven to 375°F. Cook the pasta shells according to package instructions until al dente. Drain and set aside.

2. In a large skillet, cook the ground beef over medium heat until browned and crumbled, 5-7 minutes. Drain any excess fat.

3. Add the diced onion and minced garlic to the skillet. Cook for 2-3 minutes until the onion is translucent.

4. Stir in the tomato sauce, oregano, salt, and pepper. Simmer for 5 minutes.

5. In a large bowl, mix together the ricotta cheese, 1 cup of the mozzarella cheese, the Parmesan cheese, and the beaten egg until well combined.

6. Spread 1/2 cup of the meat sauce in the bottom of a 9x13 inch baking dish.

7. Stuff each cooked pasta shell with a heaping spoonful of the ricotta cheese mixture, then place the stuffed shells in the baking dish in a single layer.

8. Pour the remaining meat sauce over the top of the stuffed shells.

9. Sprinkle the remaining 1 cup of mozzarella cheese over the top.

10. Bake the stuffed shells in the preheated oven for 25-30 minutes, until the cheese is melted and bubbly.

Serve the beef and cheese stuffed shells warm. Enjoy!

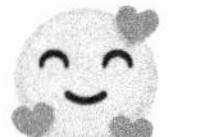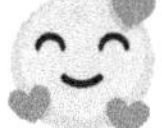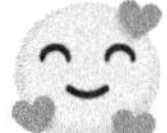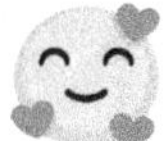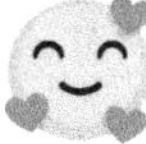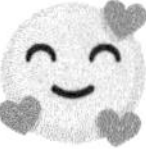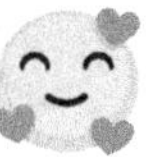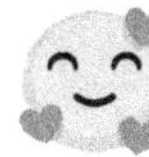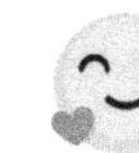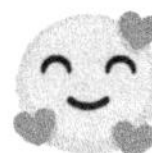

116. Buffalo chicken dip pizza

Let's do that and fill in the time here  Prep Time :    Cook Time :   Servings :

Write 5 friends with whom you want to share this dish

....
....
....
....

INGREDIENTS

- 1 lb boneless, skinless chicken breasts
- 1/2 cup buffalo sauce (such as Frank's RedHot)
- 1 (8 oz) package cream cheese, softened
- 1/2 cup ranch dressing
- 1 cup shredded cheddar cheese
- 1 (12-14 oz) pre-baked pizza crust
- 1/4 cup crumbled blue cheese (optional)
- Chopped fresh parsley for garnish (optional)

Is this dish easy or difficult for you to make?

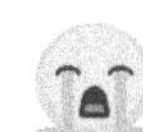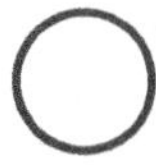 ◯   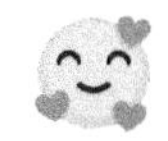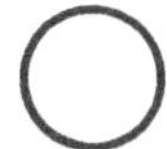 ◯

1. Preheat your oven to 400°F.

2. Place the chicken breasts in a baking dish and bake for 20-25 minutes, until cooked through. Allow to cool slightly, then shred the chicken using two forks.

3. In a medium bowl, mix together the shredded chicken, buffalo sauce, softened cream cheese, and ranch dressing until well combined.

4. Spread the buffalo chicken dip mixture evenly over the pre-baked pizza crust, leaving a small border around the edges.

5. Sprinkle the shredded cheddar cheese over the top of the dip.

6. If desired, crumble the blue cheese over the pizza as well.

7. Bake the buffalo chicken dip pizza in the preheated oven for 12-15 minutes, or until the cheese is melted and bubbly.

8. Remove the pizza from the oven and garnish with chopped fresh parsley, if desired.

9. Slice and serve the buffalo chicken dip pizza warm.

This pizza combines the flavors of classic buffalo chicken dip with a crispy pizza crust, making it a delicious and fun option for young teens. The spicy buffalo sauce, creamy dip, and melted cheese create an irresistible flavor profile.

Did you have fun cooking this dish?

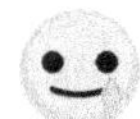 ◯   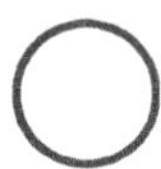 ◯

How would you rate this dish?

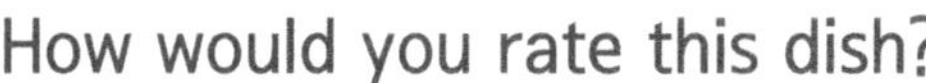
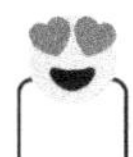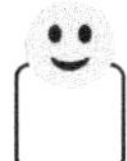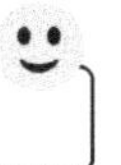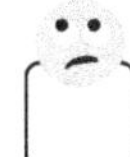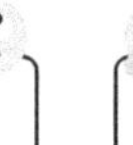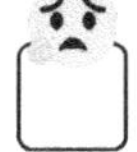

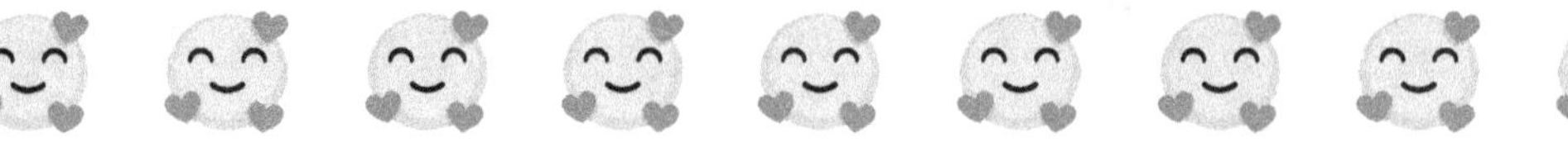

117. Cheesy bacon ranch fries

 *Let's do that and fill in the time here* **Prep Time :** 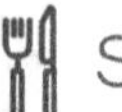 Cook Time : Servings :

Write 5 friends with whom you want to share this dish
....
....
....
....
....

INGREDIENTS

- 1 lb frozen french fries
- 6 slices bacon, cooked until crispy and crumbled
- 1 cup shredded cheddar cheese
- 1/2 cup ranch dressing
- 2 tablespoons chopped fresh parsley (optional)

Is this dish easy or difficult for you to make?

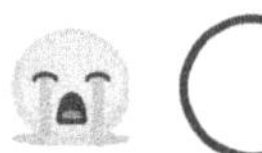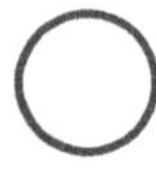 ◯   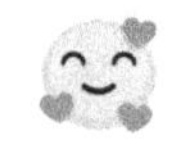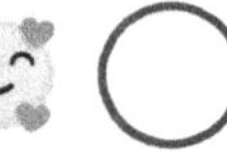 ◯

1. Preheat your oven to 425°F. Spread the frozen french fries in a single layer on a large baking sheet.

2. Bake the fries for 20-25 minutes, flipping halfway, until golden brown and crispy.

3. Remove the baked fries from the oven and top them with the crumbled bacon and shredded cheddar cheese.

4. Return the loaded fries to the oven and bake for an additional 5 minutes, until the cheese is melted and bubbly.

5. Drizzle the ranch dressing evenly over the cheesy bacon fries.

6. Sprinkle the chopped fresh parsley over the top, if desired.

7. Serve the cheesy bacon ranch fries immediately, while hot and crispy.

These loaded fries are a delicious and indulgent treat that young teens are sure to love. The combination of crispy fries, melted cheese, crispy bacon, and creamy ranch dressing is irresistible. It's the perfect snack or side dish for any occasion.

Did you have fun cooking this dish?

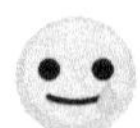 ◯   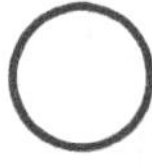 ◯

How would you rate this dish?

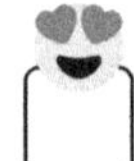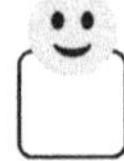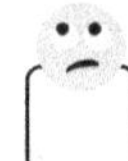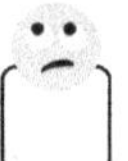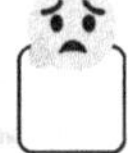

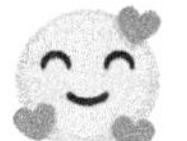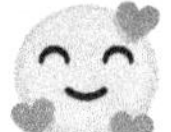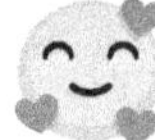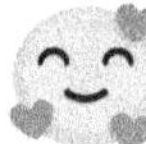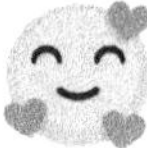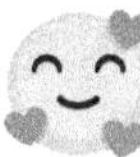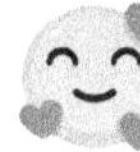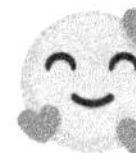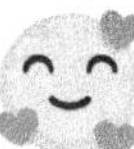

118. Chicken fajita bowl

Let's do that and fill in the time here

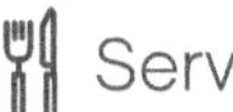 Prep Time :

Cook Time :

Servings :

Write 5 friends with whom you want to share this dish

....
....
....
....
....

Is this dish easy or difficult for you to make?

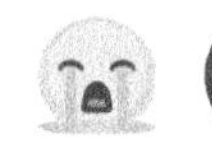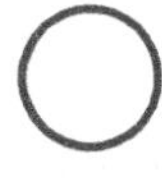 ◯   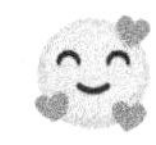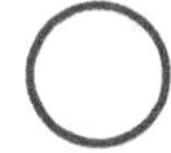 ◯

INGREDIENTS

- 1 lb boneless, skinless chicken breasts
- 2 tablespoons fajita seasoning
- 1 tablespoon olive oil
- 1 red bell pepper, sliced
- 1 green bell pepper, sliced
- 1 onion, sliced
- 2 cups cooked rice
- 1 (15 oz) can black beans, drained and rinsed
- 1 cup shredded cheddar or Monterey Jack cheese
- Toppings (optional): diced tomatoes, sliced avocado, sour cream, salsa, etc.

1. Preheat your grill or a large skillet over medium-high heat.

2. Season the chicken breasts evenly with the fajita seasoning.

3. Grill or cook the chicken in the skillet for 5-7 minutes per side, until cooked through. Allow to rest for 5 minutes, then slice or shred the chicken.

4. In the same skillet, heat the olive oil over medium-high heat. Add the sliced bell peppers and onion. Sauté for 5-7 minutes, until the vegetables are tender and slightly charred.

5. Divide the cooked rice between 4 bowls. Top each bowl with the sliced or shredded chicken, sautéed peppers and onions, black beans, and shredded cheese.

6. Finish the bowls with any desired toppings like diced tomatoes, sliced avocado, sour cream, or salsa.

This chicken fajita bowl is a fun, customizable, and nutritious meal that young teens are sure to love. The combination of the tender chicken, fresh veggies, and flavorful toppings makes for a delicious and satisfying dish.

Did you have fun cooking this dish?

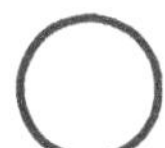 ◯   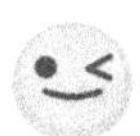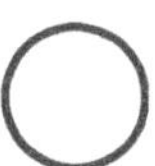 ◯

How would you rate this dish?

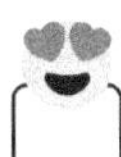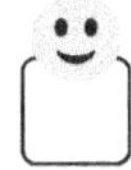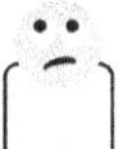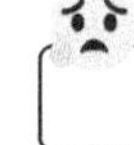

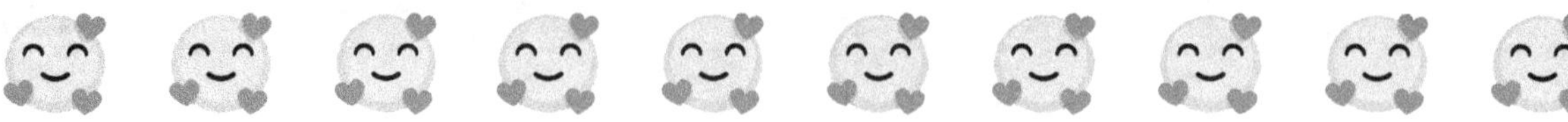

119. Beef and bean tostadas

 Prep Time :   Cook Time :   Servings :

Write 5 friends with whom you want to share this dish

Is this dish easy or difficult for you to make?

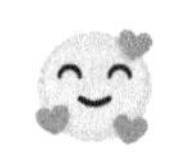 ◯   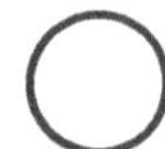 ◯

INGREDIENTS

- 1 lb ground beef
- 1 packet taco seasoning
- 1/2 cup water
- 1 (15 oz) can refried beans
- 8 pre-made tostada shells
- 1 cup shredded lettuce
- 1 cup diced tomatoes
- 1 cup shredded cheddar cheese
- Toppings (optional): sour cream, salsa, guacamole, etc.

1. In a large skillet, cook the ground beef over medium heat until browned and crumbled, about 5-7 minutes. Drain any excess fat.

2. Add the taco seasoning and water to the skillet. Stir and simmer for 2-3 minutes until the sauce thickens.

3. Spread about 2-3 tablespoons of the refried beans onto each tostada shell.

4. Top the refried beans with a heaping spoonful of the seasoned ground beef.

5. Sprinkle the shredded lettuce, diced tomatoes, and shredded cheddar cheese over the beef.

6. If desired, add any additional toppings like sour cream, salsa, or guacamole.

7. Serve the beef and bean tostadas immediately, while the shells are still crispy.

These tostadas are a fun and flavorful Mexican-inspired dish that young teens are sure to love. The combination of the crispy tostada shell, savory beef, creamy beans, and fresh toppings makes for a delicious and satisfying meal or snack.

Did you have fun cooking this dish?

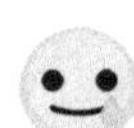 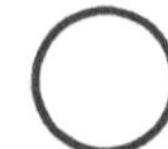 ◯   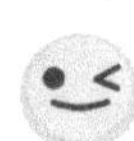 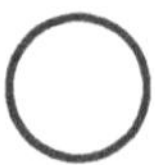 ◯

How would you rate this dish?

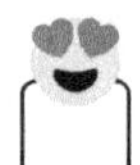 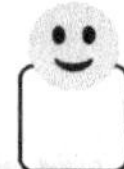 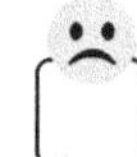 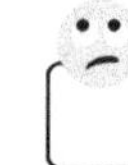 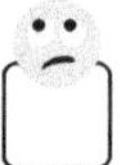 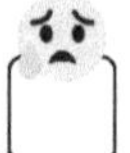

Thank You!

Dear Reader,

Thank you for choosing ***"The Complete Cookbook for Young Teens: Empower Young Chefs with Nutritious Meals and Tasty Snacks They Can Make Themselves."*** Your decision to bring this book into your home means a lot to us, and we're thrilled to be part of your culinary journey.

Cooking is a wonderful skill that not only nourishes the body but also sparks creativity and fosters independence. By investing in this cookbook, you're empowering yourself or a young chef in your life to explore the joys of cooking —whether it's whipping up a quick snack after school or preparing a family meal that brings everyone together.

We've designed this book with you in mind, offering over 100 recipes that are easy to follow, nutritious, and, above all, delicious. Each recipe is crafted to inspire confidence in the kitchen, helping you develop essential cooking techniques and a love for wholesome ingredients.

As you dive into these pages, we hope you discover new flavors, gain valuable skills, and create cherished memories around the table with loved ones. Cooking is more than just preparing food; it's about enjoying the process and sharing the joy of homemade meals with others.

Once again, thank you for your purchase. We're excited for you to embark on this culinary adventure and can't wait to see what delicious creations you'll bring to life!

Happy cooking!

Warm regards,